OBAMINABLE CARE
CARE
A Prescription For
CHAOS

By
James W. Forsythe, M.D., H.M.D.

Obaminable Care ~ A Prescription for Chaos

Century Wellness Publishing

Designed by Patty Atcheson Melton, Wow! Design Marketing

Forsythe, James W.

1. Health   2. Insurance

"I support health care for the people. I want people well taken care of. But I also want health care that we can afford as a country. I have people and friends closing down their businesses because of Obamacare."
--*Donald Trump, World-famous billionaire*

Dedication

This book is dedicated to everyone who has worked or currently works in the medical industry, and their patients.

Contents

Forward

The national and world economies and the entire medical industry are on the verge of horrific disaster due largely to the federal government's pending health care reform regulations—commonly known as "Obamacare."

Formally "The Patient Protection and Affordable Care Act," this ill-advised and misguided legislation would put a whopping 16 percent of the U.S. economy under the control of our incompetent and bureaucratic federal government. Within several years that total will grow by some accounts to a disturbing 20 percent of the economy.

To anyone who asks for my opinion on this urgent issue, I feel a need to tell them flat-out: "Unless we take decisive action to stop this process as soon as possible, extreme and difficult-to-reverse calamities will adversely impact every aspect of society."

Physicians, patients, business leaders and other people from around the world have asked me to write this book, fresh on the heels of my various successful publications, some in conjunction with media sensation Suzanne Somers,. Just as important, these many backers have urged me to help take a leadership role in fighting Obamacare.

"I have no other choice but to accept," I've told them. "To do otherwise would be to turn my back on my responsibilities as a physician and as a concerned citizen."

Now in my fifth decade as a practicing oncologist, and also a doctor of homeopathic medicine, every day I see the harm suffered by patients and medical professionals as a result of the heartless and sluggish medical insurance industry.

Exacerbating these difficulties, lawyers in today's suit-happy society have instigated frivolous, expensive and mostly unnecessary litigation. Adding even more proverbial poison to the brew, the greedy pharmaceutical industry has used high-paid lobbyists to stick its greedy paws deep into the heart of the American political process.

Seizing upon an increasing sense of urgency, the first edition of this book started rolling off printing presses less than several weeks after lawyers for and against Obamacare gave their arguments to the U.S. Supreme Court in March 20012. Most analysts predicted that the court would issue its ruling within five months by mid-summer, perhaps in June 2012.

Fully acknowledging that "time is of the essence," almost as if facing a Doomsday Clock clicking down the final seconds before midnight, I summarily vowed to update this publication as necessary when warranted by changing developments.

But why did I embrace this sense of urgency?

As you'll soon discover in more specific, concise detail on the pages that follow, a widespread medical industry disaster of gargantuan proportions faces us all unless Congress repeals Obamacare before these stifling new regulations start to click into full gear in phases within several years.

Unless we win this necessary political battle all of society will suffer seemingly irreversible physical and financial hardships for many generations to come.

Chapter 1

Obamacare Equals a Disaster of Monumental Proportions

A disaster of monumental and irreversible proportions will impact virtually all of American society if Obamacare is allowed to click into full gear.

Virtually all Americans will suffer negative impacts if this regulation becomes fully active as planned, robbing the nation of its free-enterprise system that has played a pivotal and essential role in helping to make the United States great.

Among just some of the many negative outcomes hampering the entire medical industry and consumers:

Economic collapse: First and foremost, although very few analysts have been willing to step forward and say this in no uncertain terms—the regulations could very well result in the collapse of the nation's industrial backbone and infrastructure.

Corruption: If implemented fully as planned, Obamacare is likely to spark widespread corruption on such a massive and pervasive scale that at least in some regards the Prohibition outlawing alcohol in the United States from 1919 to 1933 will pale by comparison.

Fewer doctors: Hampered by bureaucratic regulations that result in exorbitant operational costs, huge percentages of physicians will leave the industry. Worsening matters, fewer potential new doctors will be willing to enter this mindless medical industry maze sparked by the Obama administration's push for socialist-style government.

Soaring costs: The decrease in doctors will cause an unstoppable and catastrophic domino effect, resulting is sharp increases in the costs that physicians must impose upon patients in order to remain in business.

Government gimmicks: Federal and state government bureaucrats will "jerry-rig" the accounting process. The heartless and insensitive bean counters will do this largely in an effort to "cook the books," giving the deceitful appearance of supposed savings that do not actually exist.

Uninsured totals soar: Contrary to the supposed primary objective of Obamacare, the actual total number of uninsured Americans will continue to soar at least through 2019. According to the Federal Budget Office, that year the total number of uninsured people will remain at a whopping 23 million individuals.

Bureaucratic decisions: Bureaucrats who have absolutely no medical training will serve on various critical panels—making "life-and-death" decisions on whether physicians will be allowed to administer certain types of treatments.

Political favoritism: Under the primary legislation, all major corporations will have to pay health insurance for all employees—unless the companies apply for and receive exceptions. Sadly, well before the full brunt of Obamacare kicks into full gear, some huge companies are benefiting from this "crony system" while the "little guy" suffers.

Bureaucracy Will Run Amuck

Unless adversaries of Obamacare successfully repeal these new regulations in time, the entire medical industry will get bogged down in a bureaucratic maze.

For many patients, scheduling and visiting a physician to get basic check-ups or primary care will become a scheduling burden—far worse than now. And for doctors, the entire process will essentially become the equivalent of "walking on eggshells" in order to conform to stupid, idiotic government regulations.

Largely as a result, you should fully expect the non-violent war to intensify between the heartless government and the greedy insurance industry it attempt to regulate.

Think of it this way. What if you required all auto insurance companies to accept every convicted drunken driver—at rates equal to those of policy holders who have good driving records? Such a rule would seem like total lunacy, right—especially since "good drivers" would be paying more to cover their share of the burden.

Well, under its "shared responsibility" rules, Obamacare would require insurance companies to allow everyone with "pre-existing conditions"—other than smokers—to receive policies with premiums at levels equal to those of healthy people. Thus, whether the Obama administration likes to admit this or not, the vast majority of "regular people" will start paying more in health insurance than they have been.

Needless to say, as Obamacare steadily kicks into gear, the "regular guy" will get stuck with higher monthly healthy insurance bills in order to "carry the weight" of those with serious pre-existing medical conditions.

Misguided Effort Leads to Disaster

Obamacare hails as a misguided and deranged effort to strengthen and solidify the USA's medical system, largely an effort to guarantee that everyone has health insurance.

Instead, irrefutable statistics already show that the legislation is already sharply boosting health care costs while leaving many people uninsured. Worsening matters, Obamacare drastically boosts the already bloated federal bureaucracy while increasing budget deficits.

Adding insult to injury, as noted by the Heritage Foundation political action organization, the legislation "gives bureaucrats the power to influence medical decision making, which rightfully belongs in the hands of doctors and patients."

As if all this wasn't already bad enough, as the Foundation clearly states, Obamacare's "new taxes and expansion of government health care programs are unaffordable to current and future taxpayers."

Obaminable Care ~ A Prescription for Chaos

Like growing numbers of physicians and patients nationwide I fully realize that these problems mark just the beginning of a long list of challenging issues. Collectively, we're forced by these irrefutable facts to face the truth about the legislation's many failures.

Every American Will Suffer

Sadly, as my intense research on this issue clearly shows, virtually all Americans will suffer as a result of this misguided and ill-advised legislation.

These negative consequences will continue to swell in breath and scope on a massive scale unless Congress repeals Obamacare—particularly before the legislation reaches its maturity. As enacted by our nation's top elected leaders, the many various specific provisions of these foolish regulations click into gear in phases through January 1, 2018.

Whatever their own individual political ideology, all concerned Americans need to realize that the legislation got rammed through in 2010, primarily because at the time the legislation passed one political party that held the bulk of power in Washington, D.C.—the Democrats.

Whether we want to admit this or not, "bad things" are likely to happen whenever a single political party seizes the bulk of power in a democracy or a republic such as the United States. In this case, the Democratic Party held power in Congress and the White House in early 2010.

Largely as a result, the 111th United States Congress will forever be hailed as a failure. That elected body condemned future generations to bumbling bureaucratic medical regulations—unless lawmakers ultimately show the courage necessary to repeal the legislation.

Political Shenanigans Hijacked Common Sense

Over-the-top liberals rammed through the legislation despite public opinion polls clearly showing that a vast majority of Americans opposed the legislation at the time that the regulations passed. Most voters queried in recent surveys dislike Obamacare even more than a few years ago.

In passing their health care reform, the Democrats seemed to be saying: "To heck with the people. We know what's best for the public, so let's ram through this legislation in creating a nanny state. We need to tell the public which doctors they can see, when they can get treatment—and we'll appoint a panel of non-physicians to make vital decisions on life and death matters."

Whether we like to admit this or not, the fact remains that politicians made a game of the American health care system.

"Just because those politicians happened to win election, they think they have a right to play hardball with the finances and lives of everyday citizens," some analysts correctly observed. "But instead, they rammed the legislation through—recklessly and carelessly."

To their credit, all 39 Republicans in the Senate on December 24, 2009, voted against the over-the-top, ultra-liberal measure. Yet two Senators listed as independents joined their Democratic Party colleagues in passing the legislation.

On the House side of the U.S. Capitol Building, in March 2010 the bill eventually became law when representatives approved the Act by a margin of just seven—219 votes to 212. Overjoyed with the notion that his name might go down in history as an innovator on behalf of the people, President Barack Obama celebrated along with his political cronies. Rather than acting as heroes, the nation's chief executives and his "yes" people turned their backs on the needs and desires of the American people.

This Issue Transcends Party Lines

Right off the bat I feel a need to point out that I'm a registered Republican and my wife Earlene even served as the GOP's Nevada state chair early in the 21st Century.

Obamacare hails as a significant issue that should transcend party lines, no matter what our own particularly political affiliation and party preferences.

For the most part, the legislation got passed primarily for political reasons, largely because certain ultra-liberal lawmakers wanted to sharply expand the federal bureaucracy. But as I'll clearly show in the pages that follow, the Act will actually worsen problems for uninsured Americans while drastically boosting medical costs.

A primary objective of Obama and his political cronies had been to lower medical costs. Yet they quickly crafted the legislation without first "clearly analyzing" the eventual results, almost as if to quietly whisper to themselves: "We'll worry about details later."

Largely as a result, as the 2012 general election approached amid Obama's re-election campaign, his misguided medical legislation became an increasingly heated political issue.

Those within the hierarchy of the Democratic began to embrace the legislation as if it were a God's-send from heaven. Meantime, to their credit, all the remaining major Republican candidates for president through the spring vowed to make the repeal of Obamacare their top priority upon assuming office in early 2013.

Take Decisive Action Right Away

While awaiting the outcome of the U.S. Supreme Court's expected mid-summer decision on this vital issue in around June of 2012, all concerned Americans held a responsibility to take decisive action to push for repeal of Obamacare. Any failure to push for such a reversal would have to "give up too early" and accept the approaching medical industry collapse and what I fear will emerge as nationwide economic disaster. Everyone concerned about the effects of Obamacare should:

Presidency: During the 2012 general election season, support and vote for a candidate who vows to repeal Obamacare as soon as possible.

Congress: Support and vote for candidates who have the courage to say flat-out during the campaign that Obamacare is "wrong" and that it should be repealed.

I personally wish that a critical issue such as Obamacare never involved the political arena. Yet the cold truth mandates that those of us with the courage and gumption to fight the legislation should take the bold measures necessary to have the measure repealed.

Determined to push help American survive or avoid this pending crisis, I planned to spend the spring, summer and fall of 2012l encouraging everyone possible to push for the repeal of Obamacare—while also campaigning for or supporting candidates who oppose the Act.

Chapter 2

Seize the Moment for Optimal Results

Rather than sitting on our butts and "watching the political game," those of us concerned about health care should jump into this arena to champion our cause.

Certainly, Obamacare reigns as more than merely a political issue involving conservative verses liberal. In essence everything comes down to a war between common sense on the Republican side and idiocy on the Democrat hideouts.

Yes, there's no "politically correct" way to say this—Obamacare is flat-out stupid.

Thus, as I continue to spread the truth about the legislation, we should strive to convince Democrats and political independents to join in the political fight against Obamacare.

Ultimately, Obamacare is poised to rip apart the very essence of our free enterprise system. As horrific and far-fetched as this might sound, "To let Obamacare slide through unscathed would be to harm all aspects of society."

You see, if we allow the heartless federal government to dictate when and how we get our medical care, when would such lunacy end? Unless we quickly and fully eliminate this regulation as a pathway to all-out socialism, would our government eventually seek to regulate and monitor what we eat, when and how? If elected people can dictate your medical care, what's to stop them from eventually regulating how and where you spend your money—or even how you spend your free time?

"By acting under the guise as if they're trying to help us—to decide what is 'best' for us—the ultra-liberals are actually enslaving us," I tell my friends and even patients if they happen to inquire. "The liberals are busy trying to control everything about our lives, as if to say that they should make all our decisions—that they know what's best for everyone—that we should depend on them—and that we're all too stupid to make our own decisions. Well, to them I say, 'Balderdash. Keep your creepy political ideas to yourselves, and let the American people maintain their freedom."

Some Conservatives Hold Blame as Well

Whether the leaders within the Republican Party want to admit this or not, some among our ranks also hold at least some blame in failing to seize control of this vital medical-care issue.

Through the 1990s and during the first several years of this decade, the GOP watched as health care costs skyrocketed. All along the number uninsured people soared as a result, and the overall quality of medical care sagged somewhat.

At the time, as conservatives, we should have seized upon the issue and essentially "made it our own." This way, we could have crafted legislation or policies that could have helped level the proverbial playing field within the free-market medical care system.

But instead those within the Democratic Party took the primary role in quickly and recklessly crafting the Obamacare legislation. This enabled the ultra-liberals to essentially seize control of the issue, essentially becoming the first or foremost in the public mindset in "making this issue their own"—while also wrongly portraying Republicans as heartless.

To the contrary, those of us within the GOP truly care about the public's welfare, while also championing the medical industry's ability to generate reasonable profits or returns on investments.

Only this way can physicians and other medical industry professionals make the vital and necessary innovations to improve the overall quality and efficiency of health care. Meantime, a competitive playing field made possible by the elimination of Obamacare would help ensure that patient's costs remain reasonable.

Enact Sensible Legislation

Instead of merely dismantling and shredding Obamacare, the Republicans need to join with everyone including certain Democrats and Independents who all are determined to enact reasonable health care legislation.

Rather than generating a gargantuan, out-of-touch and bloated federal bureaucracy, this mandate—which I label as "Common-Sense Care" would:

Size: Limit the size of government-related bureaucracies involving health care, or more preferably ban our outlaw such agencies altogether.

Taxes: Rather than impose new taxes on certain medical-related products or services such as those imposed by Obamacare, this system would outlaw or limit such fees.

Patients: Like Obamacare, the "Common-Sense Care" system would guarantee certain rights for patients. But unlike Obamacare, Common-Sense Care would avoid placing huge, cumbersome and difficult-to-manage burdens on medical supply distributors, service providers, physicians and hospitals.

Costs: In order to help minimize costs imposed upon patients, society would encourage a competitive free-market system—rather than giving the bulk of serving options to only a handful of physicians, product manufacturers or service providers.

Bureaucratic Panels: Common-Sense Care legislation would ban or even criminalize the implementation of government-appointed panels designed to regulate the medical industry. By contrast, the Obamacare legislation reaches the point of lunacy by appointing many dozens of panels or committees. For the most part, many of these bodies are comprised of bean counters and bureaucrats who have absolutely no knowledge whatsoever of medicine or treatments.

Free Enterprise Systems: Common-Sense Care will clear the

James W. Forsythe, M.D., H.M.D.

way for the vital and essential free-market competitive system. Such a program will clear the way for researchers, entrepreneurs and pharmaceutical companies to generate all-new, unique and cutting-edge technology, medicines and treatments.

Unfettered and unencumbered by bureaucratic federal regulations, medical industry professionals under my plan would be free to passionately research diseases—and ultimately develop cures. This, in turn, would result in more choices for consumers in a competitive environment, lowering or at least minimize doctor-related expenses.

By contrast, the Obamacare infrastructure literally bogs down the essential free-market system—thereby making the implementation of urgent medical industry advancements almost impossible. Investors would be reluctant to give resources to innovators, fearful that crappy and unnecessary government regulations would stifle or even end their efforts—while also lessening the potential for profitability.

All Government Medical Reforms Have Failed

Even amid the earliest years of its implementation, Obamacare marks just the latest in a long list of failed efforts by the federal government to overhaul the medical industry.

One of the most notable "failures" or misguided attempts came in the early 1990s, during the first term of the Clinton Administration.

President Bill Clinton made the ill-advised decision of appointing his wife, First Lady Hillary Rodham Clinton, to oversee efforts to enact health care reform.

According to many historians and political observers, overall the Clintons' effort evolved into a dismal disaster. Like Obamacare, the Clinton plans strived to essentially grow into an "everything to everyone, help everyone" plan.

Ultimately, the Clinton effort became an unworkable hodge-podge crammed with political correctness—essentially identical, at least in that regard, to Obamacare.

Obaminable Care ~ A Prescription for Chaos

Like Barack Obama eventually would during the first year of his administration, shortly after taking office Bill Clinton strived to create some sort of huge legislation that would embolden his name and legacy for many generations or centuries to come.

Perhaps Obama feared that without his own deranged medical reform plan, through the passage of time his administration or presidential accomplishments would simply fade into obscurity—other than being known as the first president "of color."

But sadly, in a rush to gain enduring political fame, within less than one year after first taking office Obama started pushing through his medical industry reform legislation. Overly rushed to create a legacy for himself, Obama started ramming through his proposal without first setting a solid, reasonable framework for such legislation.

Political Hogwash Won the Day

Even those of us who embrace an opposing ideology often admit that President Obama possesses vastly superior oratory skills as compared to many of his political adversaries.

Sure enough, through his efforts to push Obamacare throughout 2009 and into early 2010, the president essentially told the public what they wanted to hear.

First, he promised that people who already had insurance that they liked would be able to continue to visit their favorite physicians.

And, either intentionally deceiving the public or woefully ignorant of his own plan's many failings, Obama also insisted that his sweeping medical industry legislation would hold down health care costs. Just as important, he strived to assure the public that his safety net would make medical coverage affordable and available to everyone.

To the contrary, well before the full force of Obamacare clicks into gear, the president's legislation had already dismally failed in virtually every regard.

Nonetheless, Obama's proposals came at what some political

observers perceived as an ideal time, when many major medical insurance companies faced extreme financial difficulties and as millions of people lacked funds for health insurance. Continually increasing medical coverage fees made such policies unaffordable for many Americans.

Obamacare Became a Dismal Failure

As clearly documented by many clear-minded, unbiased observers, Obamacare started flopping in almost every regard almost right away. Among those adversely impacted according to continually updated findings of the Heritage Foundation:

Seniors: "Nearly one quarter of all seniors rely on Medicare Advantage, the private health care option in Medicare. However, Obamacare makes such deep cuts to that program that half of those covered will no longer be able to keep the coverage that they have." Compounding this problem, the Foundation says, at least $47 billion in new taxes Obamacare imposes on drug companies and medical device makers—along with new reporting requirements and regulations imposed on physicians—"will make access to health care and services more costly for seniors."

Doctors: While Obamacare floods the medical industry with 18 million more people added to the Medicaid program, physicians will be reimbursed for only "56 percent of the market rate for medical procedures." Worsening this situation further, as noted by the Foundation, "due to increased regulation and less reimbursement, 65 percent of doctors are considering no longer accepting government health programs."

Business and the Economy: Small and medium-size companies will get slapped with a maze of fees and government-mandated regulations. Many business executives now acknowledge that these rules will prevent them from expanding their operations or adding new employees—thereby severely damaging an already fragile national economy that depends on growth. As if pushing a platinum dagger clear the heart of American industry, Obamacare will slap businesses with $52 billion in taxes requiring that employers provide health insurance. As noted by the Foundation, on February 10, 2011, Congressional Budget Office Director Doug Elmendorf testified that Obamacare will result in an estimated 800,000 fewer U.S. jobs.

U.S. state governments: Mandates enforced by Obamacare will collectively force state governments nationwide to collectively fork out many tens of billions of dollars toward Medicaid. The size and significance of this challenge comes into focus when taking into account that more than 80 million people will be on Medicaid by 2019. This in turn will force already-strapped taxpayers to foot the bills. These inexcusably high costs left at least 21 states Attorneys General with no choice other than to file a suit seeking to protect their citizens from being forced to pay for such nonsense.

Future Generations and Families: The Foundation reports that Obamacare "adds a trillion dollars in new health care spending." The organization's experts report that this expands prohibitively expensive entitlements and creates a "subsidy scheme that discourages work and penalizes marriage."

President Obama Gave Unfulfilled Promises

All these many difficulties mark just the tip of the proverbial iceberg that encompasses the upcoming bureaucratic nightmare. In fact, even the bureaucrats with the Obama administration acknowledge that the 2,400-page legislation will woefully fail to deliver the president's promised benefits to American society and to individual citizens.

Courageous and stepping up in support of a more common-sense approach, through 2011 various citizens groups and local governments nationwide launched efforts to legally fight this reckless and debilitating legislation.

In Florida, for instance, several state legislators pushed for statewide regulations that would prohibit the enforcement of any laws that would require buying health insurance. Some analysts initially labeled such efforts as meaningless, since federal regulations effectively "trump state laws."

Nevertheless, some observers viewed various similar efforts in Florida and other states as a significant stride in blocking any potential future attempts to form individual state-operated mandatory health insurance programs such as regulations in Massachusetts.

According to news reports, in the early spring of 2012 various Catholic organizations in several states banded together to protest Obamacare. Meantime, courageous officials in several states— primarily Republicans—continued their individual and regional efforts to wipe out Obamacare in state and local courts.

As the propaganda war intensified to a fever pitch, catchy anti-Obamacare quotes began to riddle the Internet. Among my personal favorites are "Pay the Government or Die," and my own creative phrase used as inspiration for the title of this book—"Obaminable Care."

Obamacare is Worse Than the Famed Abominable Snowman

The Obamacare legislation and the famous ice monster the Abominable Snowman can be easily compared. A frightening picture soon erupts amid such analysis when we soon realize that the federal legislation is far worse than a monster in a B-grade 1950s horror movie.

Legends and age-old mythology designates the "abominable snowman" as an ape-like creature that inhabits the Tibetan and Himalayan regions. Sometimes called "Yeti," this horrific and dangerous creature is translated as "man-bear" in some literature.

Like the Obamacare program, the snowman's dangers and evil-minded focus is often difficult for an average uninformed person to detect or sense. Some translations even go so far as to refer to the snowman as "filthy"—thus resulting in the word "abominable."

Like the monstrous snowman, Obamacare is unclean, untested

and highly dangerous to all of society. Mirroring the snowman, Obamacare is wild, untamed and capable of literally mowing down and freezing up everyone in its path—both friend and foe.

Learn How This Monstrous Legislation Impacts Your Family

Following intense research on this issue for several years, I have concluded that if left unchecked Obamacare will have an adverse impact on virtually all American families. Although sociologists insist that for the most part "nothing should be considered as average," here is what you can and should expect as a result of the legislation:

Jobs: If you're an unemployed adult right now, your chances of finding a good, long-term job will decrease markedly. Soaring costs coupled with cumbersome government mandates will force many employers to cut back on workforce totals, lessening your chances of finding solid employment.

Business: Small businesses will close at an alarming rate, unable to afford the mandated costs and bureaucratic oversights. This in turn will permanently cripple the U.S. economy, forcing major employers to move more jobs overseas—perhaps even more positions than were eliminated from the late 1980s through the first decade of this century.

Incomes: The average person's per-capita spending income will decrease sharply, as legislation forces employers to push higher percentages of their limited financial resources to Obamacare-related bureaucratic expenditures.

Crime: As previously indicated, behind-the-scenes white collar crime will increase sharply, as some unscrupulous employers strive to "cook the books" in an effort to avoid ludicrous Obamacare related taxes and regulations.

Bureaucracy: The federal bureaucracy will turn "upside down" in economic terms, with the overall non-government economy producing less in terms of financial capital than elected officials will need to operate the government.

Economic crash: The burdensome infrastructure coupled with swelling federal budget deficits totaling "tens of trillions of dollars" will eventually result in a catastrophic economic collapse—which will make the Great Depression of the 1930s pale by comparison.

Beware if Obamacare Becomes Entrenched

When and if Obamacare goes into full force and becomes entrenched in the USA's culture, many of us who oppose the legislation fear "there will be no turning back."

Just like with Medicaid, Medicare and Social Security, once the American people get a federal entitlement our citizenry is likely to "want it forever." In essence, unless we take decisive action to stop Obamacare now, people eventually will think of themselves as entitled to those services from the cradle to the grave.

This in effect will come as a recipe for disaster, since when and if the legislation clicks into full gear it'll be so huge and cumbersome that little if anything can fix or curtail the resulting problems.

Picture the situation this way. In essence, as a society we're collectively halfway up a hill. The vast majority of us agreed that something needed to be done to fix health care.

But up above us the makings of Obamacare started amassing at the top of the hill. This will gradually build up and cascade downward as if an unstoppable and highly predictable avalanche destined to cover and smother us all.

At this juncture, the only reliable way to prevent the inevitable damage is to virtually stop Obamacare in its tracks. The best method for achieving this is through political action, although the ultra-liberal coalition holds up a formidable roadblock.

Chapter 3

I Went Into Mourning at Election Time

A deep and foreboding depression struck me on the day after the American people first elected Barack Obama to the presidency in November 2008.

Every fiber of my being, the essence of my spirit and logic told me that this man's ultra-liberal politics would destroy the American medical and health insurance systems.

During the first several days after the election, as a show of mourning and protest I wore a black arm band to my medical offices. From that day forward, I began warning my patients and other medical professions of the upcoming damage.

Sure enough, just as I had feared, shortly after assuming the presidency in early 2009 Obama went on a rampage destined to destroy and obliterate the medical industry.

From my personal perspective, this man and his devilishly liberal allies were dead-set on ramming through Obamacare for their own political glory despite its many obvious failings.

Liberals Reached the Point of Lunacy

Like many of my patients and medical industry colleagues, I cringe at the sight of old TV news clips chronicling a 2010 speech by then-Speaker of the House Nancy Pelosi. She tells an audience: "We have to pass the (Obamacare) bill so that you can find out what is in it, away from the fog of the controversy."

James W. Forsythe, M.D., H.M.D.

Yes, following the lead and guidance of liberal attack dogs such as Pelosi, in late 2009 and early 2010 the Democratic Congress rushed to pass the Patient Protection and Affordable Care Act at lightning speed—before the public could have time to react to the proposal's failings.

Adding insult to injury, as the 2012 election was just starting to kick into full gear, Pelosi had the audacity to use fear-mongering to shut down adversaries. She claimed that repealing Obamacare would cost the country 300,000 jobs.

To the contrary, however, as my research shows, to allow the medical reform rules to slide into full force unscathed could cost far more jobs—perhaps millions.

So, I say: "Shame on politicians such as Pelosi, who use lingual hogwash and scare tactics to push forth their own misguided political agendas. Such smoke-and-mirror tactics never will work in fooling me or many other dedicated physicians and their patients."

Average People Need Political Gumption

Sadly, at least judging by my many conversations with doctors and patients, huge percentages of people across the USA fail to realize the many dangers of Obamacare.

For the most part, the "average Joes and average Janes" of our nation are far too busy just struggling to survive to grasp, understand or realize the dangers of this legislation.

Worsening matters, huge sections of the public hear only bits and pieces, smatterings of sound-bites about this important issue. Steeped in political hyperbole, some whacko leftists proclaim Obamacare as the savior of Americans seeking affordable health care.

I fear that such deceptive tactics may have worked at least somewhat in fooling at least some of the public. Many average citizens lacked the time, motivation and know-how to study and analyze the legislation's complex details—let alone to enter the political fray in seeking repeal of the measure.

29

Obaminable Care ~ A Prescription for Chaos

As many of us clearly remember from history lessons, the late President Franklin Delano Roosevelt, commonly known as simply "FDR," once famously proclaimed that "the only thing we have to fear is fear itself." Well, during the current era two words should be added to the end of that famous linke: "And Obamacare."

I Quickly Chose to Take a Leadership Role

Filled with a sense of duty to my patients and to the medical profession, I felt motivated enough to take a leadership role in this political fight against Obamacare. To do otherwise would be to shun my responsibility as a doctor and as a citizen.

Since childhood, I have fully embraced the Biblical teaching of Matthew 22:14: "Many are called, but few are chosen."

At least in part I used this as a sign when entering the medical profession in the early 1960s, and later that decade when serving our country as an Army officer leading military medical teams in the Vietnam War. My inner burning sense of duty, honor and country carried over for several decades that followed, while serving as an officer—eventually a colonel—in the Army National Guard.

Some people might believe that I have already done enough to serve our country. But now in my mid-70s, I feel motivated once again by an urgent and pressing need to go into service.

This time, I have chosen to answer the call of those urging me to help take a decisive front-and-center role in doing what I legally can to help stop Obamacare dead in its tracks.

The Hate-Mongers Will Try to Suppress This Message

Now that I have achieved at least some degree of recognition within the medical industry, I know full well that many liberal detractors will strive to muddy my message.

You see, those on the extreme left would like nothing more than to rob me and others who oppose Obamacare of our freedom of speech.

My detractors in this regard, the supporters of Obamacare, might seek to tell you that I do not know what I'm talking about—that my facts are "all screwed up on this issue."

Well, to them I might say that unlike many of my detractors, I have many decades of intense experience within the heart of the American medical system. I've interacted with many dozens or hundreds of insurance companies, while personally serving the medical care needs of literally tens of thousands of patients.

I've worked first-hand and interacted with literally many diverse people, medical industry professionals and physicians. Along the way I've dealt with critical issues ranging from medical insurance payment issues through the late 20th century, to helping to implement significant advancements in patient care.

Ultimately, unlike the uninformed people who support Obamacare, I fully understand the needs and challenges of patients and physicians. When all is said and done, I know without any reservation or hesitation whatsoever that Obamacare is wrong for America—it's wrong for our people, wrong for our patients, wrong for doctors and wrong for the entire medical industry as well.

Widespread Ramifications Impact Patients

Every week patients from across the United States and around the world travel to my West Coast clinic for preventative care or treatments for cancer or other ailments.

With steadily increasing frequency many of them are asking me for my opinion on Obamacare, the medical industry in general and overall advances in treatments.

First, I tell them the good news, that for the most part physicians and medical professionals have made significant strides in developing effective treatments for a wide variety of ailments as overall life expectancies increase.

Even so, I refrain from sugar-coating my analysis. Instead, if often give no-holds-barred warnings about the precarious state of the medical industry primarily due to Obamacare.

Obaminable Care ~ A Prescription for Chaos

Of course, the direct care of my patients and implementation of their good-health regimes remains my primary focus and concern. Yet for those who take the first initiative to ask, I make no attempt whatsoever to withhold my opinion on the urgent need to repeal Obamacare as soon as possible.

Take Politics Out of This Vital Issue

In the best of all worlds, under a utopian situation and even amid today's heated philosophical debates, we all need to take politics out of the health care picture.

Ideally, from the eyes of the overall public, this should not be viewed as a Republican-verses-Democrat issue. By labeling the problem as a confrontation between liberals and conservatives, we lose sight of the vital big picture.

Ultimately, everything comes down to the fact that Obamacare is: burdensome and expensive; impossible to adequately administer; and harmful to the overall health of the economy—while robbing seniors and families of the right to make their own choices.

Rather than putting our individual and collective fates in the hands of the federal government, we should enact, embrace and appreciate a system that gives all Americans a right to exercise personal freedoms in their own health care decisions.

All along, we need to strive with great focus and unbending determination to fight against and ultimately outlaw any system such as Obamacare that imposes burdensome regulations plus crippling taxation on a single vital industry—medical care.

Watch Me Eagerly Hold Our Banner High

Without any reservation whatsoever, at the urging of my patients, friends and colleagues I have chosen to work diligently to bring this message to the forefront.

During the months immediately before the 2012 general election, and even afterward if necessary, I will work as efficiently as possible to bring this message to the people.

Called into action, whenever asked I will be making a wide variety of public presentations on this pressing issue, via TV, radio, Web conferences and medical industry seminars.

All this clicks into full gear as I reach a time in life when many people in my particular position might eagerly expect to enjoy retirement.

Yet rather than settle into a life of leisure, I'm more eager than ever to serve my steadily growing numbers of patients—while also teaching the public about Obamacare.

This is my life's calling, to assist and treat patients as a physician, while also striving to teach people about ideal medical care reform and to take a leadership role on the issue.

William Shakespeare Would Turn a Perfect Phrase

As many of us learned in high school or college, the legendary bard William Shakespeare's many famous quotes include: "Something is rotten in the state of Denmark"—from Act 1 of the timeless classic "Hamlet."

In essence, this line uttered by the lesser-known character Marcellus essentially signifies that an entire political system is rotting from its head to the core.

Well, despite what his political allies might proclaim, the same goes for the overall status of the Obama administration's continued push for his medical industry reform.

And, until those of us with the willingness, the energy and the gumption to fight and win this political battle eventually persevere, the governmental stench will continue unabated.

Taking this overall assessment even further, I'm perhaps far more critical of the current state of the medical industry than many other anti-Obamacare advocates.

Chapter 4
Problems Inflict the Overall Medical Industry

While stopping short of proclaiming that the medical profession is corrupt, I still find myself proclaiming that serious issues exist— even without Obamacare.

Perhaps the most nagging and perplexing problem is the selfishness and greed of huge pharmaceutical companies, sometimes labeled as "Big Pharma."

The world's largest drug manufacturing and pharmaceutical distribution companies, primarily based in the United States, grossly overcharge the public. Worsening the situation, these same monopolies hold undue influence over Congress due to huge campaign donations coupled with high-paid lobbyists who benefit from seemingly unstoppable access to federal lawmakers.

Compounding these problems, the U.S. Federal Food and Drug Administration, commonly known as the FDA, essentially serves as a lap dog or crony of the world's largest medical corporations and Big Pharma.

Even before the advent of Obamacare, all these factors tied together in crippling consumers, in some instances blocking them from access to effective but far less expensive remedies prescribed by practitioners of homeopathic or natural medicines.

My Professional Position Stands as Unique

To help put the overall challenge into perspective, I believe that it's important for you to know that I'm one of a handful of practicing integrative medical oncologists in the United States. As a physician specializing in the treatment and prevention of cancers and other diseases, I practice so-called standard allopathic medicine. Many Americans consider this as "regular mainstream medicine."

In addition, I also practice homeopathic medicine that concentrates largely on natural remedies rather than common, expensive "manufactured drugs."

At least to some degree, my decision to simultaneously practice both types of medicine has sparked the ire of many so-called mainstream physicians. Lots of regular doctors who view natural remedies as "quackery" dislike the fact that I often prescribe inexpensive, natural substances rather than high-priced pharmaceuticals.

Largely as a result, I have a broad perspective of the many flaws within the Obamacare organizational flow. For the most part, the overall mainstream Big Pharma industry is already inept, greedy and somewhat corrupt.

The onset and eventual implementation of Obamacare would only serve to exacerbate and weaken the overall pharmaceutical and medical system even more.

Consumer Costs Will Skyrocket Under Obamacare

Even before the full-force of Obamacare, some pharmaceutical companies are charging at least $10 or even much more for certain individual pills that patients need.

Those who support Obamacare will tell the public that these excessive, monopolistic fees will decrease thanks to the medical industry reform legislation.

My heart aches with the realization that these people have been fooled into believing such hogwash. You see, my research into the issue indicates that large drug companies will use the bureaucratic entanglements caused by Obamacare as an excuse to raise prices.

Add to this the fact that the president's plan robs consumers of the abilities to make many of their personal health care choices, and we have a recipe for financial disaster.

Obaminable Care ~ A Prescription for Chaos

Locked in collusion with the corrupt and incompetent FDA, Big Pharma is likely to use the confusion and bureaucracy to lock in excessively high drug prices.

When that happens, those who support the overly liberal policies will seek to place all blame solely on the drug companies. But the burdensome and excessively high prices will become possible and prevalent largely as a result of Obamacare.

All Citizens Need to Take Decisive Action

Throughout my campaign to repeal Obamacare, joining forces with those who feel the same, I'll be stressing strategies that all of us should take to win this essential political fight. As soon as possible, you should implement all of these tactics:

Petition: Sign an online petition showing your opposition to Obamacare. You can access the petition via at this independent political action Website, PresidentBarackHusseinObama.com

Communicate: Write, fax, email or call the offices of your state's current U.S. senators, plus the office of your congressional representative. You can find links accessing that contact information via my Website.

Book: Purchase copies of this book for your friends, associates or anyone who could benefit from learning about this issue. Make your purchases online via my political Website or directly to the Amazon.com purchase page at ObaminableCare.com

Candidates: In the 2012 general election, support presidential, congressional and statewide candidates who vow to repeal Obamacare as soon as possible. Choose what you consider the best candidates, either from the Republican or Democrat parties—as long as they're committed to eliminating Obamacare. Your support can range from campaign contributions to walking door-to-door distributing literature and displaying bumper stickers or even hosting meet-the-candidate rallies at your home or at a community building.

Blogs and Websites: Start your own personal Website or blogs opposing Obamacare, or post on other existing blogs giving your opinion.

Posters, Yard Signs and Bumper Stickers: Install these wherever you legally can. If your personal funds are limited, inquire where and how you can receive them at no charge from various local, state or national political action organizations.

Remain Vigilant at All Times

Remain persistent and relentless in carrying on this political battle, even past the United States Supreme Court's anticipated ruling in the summer of 2012 and after the fall elections. Remember, our ultra-liberal political adversaries are likely to remain steadfast in their efforts to oppose us without letup.

Everything comes down to an "information war." Our opponents are likely to use propaganda, distorting the facts in order to keep ramming through their agenda.

On the positive side, we will not need to distort the facts in order to make the public realize the truth. Nonetheless, our challenge hinges largely on our ability to convince the public that repealing Obamacare remains in their best interests.

All along, however, because the overall issue remains highly complex for the ultimate winner in this political war "the devil is in the details."

Herein emerges our primary, formidable challenge. Most people lack the time, energy or motivation to study the Obamacare issue in-depth before forming their own opinions. Fully aware of this, the pro-Obamacare forces are likely to spin the issue, proclaiming that the measure is great for the public.

All along, the proponents will falsely and ignorantly proclaim that those of us who oppose Obamacare are merely greedy people or organizations striving to continue gouging consumers on behalf of huge corporations.

We Win Public Opinion Polls

Thankfully, a wide variety of continuous polls of public opinion show that a majority of Americans have consistently opposed Obamacare.

In essence, this means that most Americans of voting age realize that this health care reform was rammed into law without their consent or support.

Public opinion polls taken at least every few weeks over the past several years show that a majority of citizens have consistently opposed Obamacare—except for on one occasion in late April of 2011 when opposition dipped to 47 percent of those surveyed.

At all other times, according to the Rasmussen Reports postings, from 50 percent to about 60 percent of those surveyed opposed Obamacare. And, on several occasions the percentage of opponents even edged above 60 percent.

From my view, anti-Obamacare advocates should use this data to push our effort forward. We need to tell voters flat-out: "The majority of the public has consistently opposed Obamacare, but its proponents are striving to ram the effort down your throats anyway. Well, the liberal need to know that we're not that stupid. And they need to allow us to retain the right and the opportunity to legally obliterate Obamacare. People who push for a bureaucratic nanny state are nothing but cruel and heartless ideologues."

Demonize Our Adversaries

In order to persevere and emerge victorious, we can and should work to demonize Obamacare supporters in the eyes of the American public.

If you consider such a tactic as raunchy, childish and cruel, keep in mind that at all times that politics is a grimy, dirty and stinky business. We've already learned that those who support this medical industry reform have strived to portray us as either ignorant or pro-Big Business monsters that will stop at nothing to financially stick it to the public.

38

Yes, just like in actual war where nations strive to dehumanize enemies in the eyes of their citizens, within the political realm skullduggery and deception reigns.

So, we should take pity on those within the 40 percent to 50 percent range of the American public who now oppose any repeal of Obamacare.

From my personal view, the vast majority of these individuals have either been hoodwinked into supporting the reform—or they fail to comprehend the facts.

Anticipate a Deceptive Show

Since he's running unopposed by any significant big-name as his party's presidential nominee, Obama will appear in early September of 2012 at the Democratic National Convention in Charlotte, North Carolina. From the view of many political analysts, this will emerge as merely a boring, highly scripted "coronation" or show—essentially free media publicity for his campaign.

Striving to take advantage of the extensive national and international news coverage, the Democrats are likely to produce a feel-good movie or media presentation—on the verge of portraying Obama as a saint.

All this, of course, will be used to "spin" the issues. This propaganda material will portray Obama in a bright light, striving to portray him and his Obamacare as if sent from heaven above.

Along with many other anti-Obamacare advocates, I fear that any Americans who take the time to watch this proverbial circus act will bite hard on the bait.

So, throughout the summer, I'll be warning people from coast to coast to refrain from falling for the sappy-sweet pro-Obama motion picture collage.

"Don't be fooled by the hogwash presented by the Obama supporters," I will tell Web surfers, TV viewers, radio listeners, Webinar participants and people at various medical industry conventions. "Avoid falling into their web of deceit."

Expect Many People to be Fooled

As this political battle intensifies, those of us who oppose Obamacare need to face the fact that many Americans likely will be fooled—sucked up into believing the president's hogwash.

Worsening matters, as I've already noted, almost every seasoned political analyst from both primary political parties acknowledges that Obama is a highly gifted, compelling orator.

Without question, the president's speaking skills have been rated as among the best of the current era, whether we like to admit this or not.

This leaves me with the realization that lots of Americans are likely to get "conned" by Obama's campaign rhetoric. Certainly he pulled off a big deceptive grand slam in the 2008 campaign when babbling about "hope" and political transparency.

Topping all this off, Obama is a highly skilled and crafty debater. During the 2008 campaign, he scored relatively well overall in a stream of debates with then-rival candidate Hillary Clinton—and eventually that year's Republican nominee, Sen. John McCain of Arizona.

Ultimately, despite these various strong points in Obama's favor, those of us opposing his medical reform have our own magic weapon—namely "the facts."

Generate Factual "Propaganda"

As a Christian and a man of great faith, I fully embrace and adhere to the Bible's John 8:32, which says: "You shall know the truth, and the truth shall set you free." A wide variety of biblical interpretations all reach similar conclusions.

Sure enough, even many agnostic people realize that the "facts speak for themselves." This way, once we present the details about Obamacare to the American public in a lively, compelling and easy-to-understand manner, we can emerge as victorious.

Largely for this reason, as they prepare for their party's

2012 National Convention in Tampa, Florida, I'm encouraging Republicans to seize that opportunity to present the many negatives about Obamacare in a compelling and emotional manner. Among key factors that I'll be recommending throughout the summer:

Film: At the convention, show a film fully dedicated to the horrors of Obamacare. Depict streams of "real" people ranging from doctors to very young and maturing patients. Accurately and fully depict how Obamacare is already wreaking havoc on their lives, causing difficulties and financial hardships, while robbing them of the ability to make vital and necessary choices about their own health care.

Consistency: Throughout the convention, have most speakers mention the horrors and ravages of Obamacare to the nation and to individuals and their families.

Acceptance speech: During his acceptance speech, the eventual nominee should spend a sizable block of time warning Americans of Obamacare's destructive path—while also honestly vowing to repeal the regulation.

Humanize stories: Largely to counter-balance the expected line of bull from Democrats at their convention the following week, the various films, images and presentations produced by Republicans need to describe or chronicle honest, heart-felt, real-live and compelling situations.

Blitz the Campaign Season

Our advertising message throughout the campaign needs to remain strong, persistent and consistent—relentlessly driving home the many faults of Obamacare.

For such a strategy to become effective, individually and collectively we need to dedicate our financial resources toward effective advertising on a national, state and regional scale. Various political analysts and advisors have been telling me that in order to generate the greatest effectiveness, this should be done on a variety of fronts.

Obaminable Care ~ A Prescription for Chaos

While many seasoned political advocates proclaim that, "All politics is local," we must illicit the help of doctors, their patients and medical professionals from virtually every state and major city—plus small towns.

Rather than merely throwing money toward blanket advertising, we must always convey a consistent theme—namely that "Obamacare does not work; it will bankrupt America; and it'll rob people of their decision-making abilities while increasing the costs of drugs, physicians visits, hospitalizations and overall medical care.

Another key necessary factor crafted into our messages should involve fear. Rather than "fear-mongering," the process of sparking unnecessary or unwarranted worries, we need to let the facts do the arguing for us. You see, at least according to many analysts, almost nothing drives people to the polls with more urgency than fear—oftentimes worries that the government or big business will rip them off, stealing from them.

Chapter 5

Danger Looms:
A Third-Party Candidate

There remains a danger that an unexpected third-party candidate could break out from the pack and enter the presidential campaign.

Such a scenario likely would emerge as a crippling blow to any anti-Obamacare effort, particularly if the candidate is a big-name conservative. Such a candidacy likely would split the anti-liberal ballot, leaving the lion's share of essential presidential Electoral College votes for Obama.

Certainly such a development would generate joyful cheers among the Democrats. In fact, I would not be surprised if liberals strive to pull such shenanigans.

In essence, pro-Obamacare supporters would be striving to take advantage of current widespread public discontent among the electorate. This way, the Democrats would strive to benefit from moderates or non-partisan voters disenchanted with the political process.

At least judging by some public opinion polls, the nation's approval rating of Congress dipped in late 2011—matching a previous all-time low. This came as particularly troubling news to the GOP, because overall Republicans garnered a higher disapproval rating than their Democrat counterparts.

Meantime, various news reports indicated that some conservative presidential candidates such as Congressman Ron Paul—a darling of the Tea Party—could break out in the late spring or summer to form an independent presidential bid.

I fear that this would essentially crack the conservative vote down the middle, pulling away vital and necessary support to the eventual Republican presidential nominee. Following a consistent trend of the past few decades, a wide variety of little-known political organizations plan to enter the race—invariably garnering little attention.

The real danger would emerge if a "big, famous name—a household name" suddenly enters the race. Please remember that this assumption discounts celebrities popular in their own specific areas of entertainment, but who lack respect or solid credentials in the political arena.

Such notables include former network TV sitcom star Rosanne Barr, a Hawaii resident who has announced her intention to run for president representing the Green Party. The many less-popular political organizations include the Libertarian Party to the Party for Socialism and Liberation.

Barr and the nominees from a hodgepodge of organizations, perhaps perceived by most voters as non-viable, would stand little chance of tipping the election either way—unless one of them recruits a highly respected media superstar.

Normally, these various political parties or ideologies would not be noteworthy enough to mention in any discussion of Obamacare. But such entities could very well play a significant role if a big-name candidate suddenly gets such a nomination.

Blast the Third Candidate

Eager to legally push Obama out of office, anti-Obamacare advocates need to immediately and soundly blast the credentials of any formidable third-party 2012 presidential candidate.

To do otherwise would be to essential bow to defeat forevermore on the grand scale of any hope of shooting down Obamacare—at least in one sudden, all-encompassing swoop.

When and if such a lion should enter the arena, as Obamacare opponents we need to collectively remain strong and focused in our efforts.

After all, the long-term well being of the American medical

industry and of patients as well could very well depend on the success or failure of our political efforts.

Within this vein, we shall never cave in to the age-old adage, "if you cannot beat them, join them." To the contrary, I shall always remain among those who will never cave in amid this philosophical fight.

Attack, Attack, Attack

We need to become vicious attack dogs in the political sense, fully cognizant at all times that the general public votes on far more than a single issue.

Embracing this strategy, those of us determined to legally take down Obama should treat this all-out political war as a ferocious arena that has no recognizable rules. Carrying this strategy to the end-game stage, we must:

Image: Convey a clear, distinct and hard-to-deny message that Obama deserves the image of someone who lacks any strong leadership skills. Let us portray him as weak-willed, essentially the leader of a rudderless ship for appointing political cronies whose whacky political philosophies fall way too far to the left—well past the philosophical limits that average Americans are willing to tolerate.

Deficit: Every step of the way, we should emphasize the undeniable fact that the federal budget deficit skyrocketed under the Obama administration. There's no end in sight to the overall budget overruns, exceeding $15.5 trillion by many accounts and still growing.

Gasoline and energy: Let's drive home the point that this guy has done virtually nothing to curtail the upward-spiraling energy costs. As voters make their final choices of who to vote for, we need to emphasize that gasoline prices are peaking at all-time highs.

Approval ratings: A wide variety of public opinion polls including the Rasmussen Reports indicate that Obama had in the spring of 2012 a negative approval rating—perhaps the lowest since

President Jimmy Carter, a one-term Democrat of the late 1970s. Even so, nearly half or about 49 percent of voters approved at least somewhat of Obama's job performance, according to Rasmussen. Even so, at least according to this one particular polling service, 14 percent more people strongly disapproved of Obama's performance than approved of him. Seizing this as an opportunity, we need to drive home to voters the fact that Obama has a high disapproval rating.

Chapter 6

Enter a Wild Card ~ The Supreme Court Ruling

Win or lose within the legal arena, the much-anticipated summer ruling on the Obamacare issue by the U.S. Supreme Court will throw a major wild card into the mix.

For the most part, at least according to my research from a wide variety of sources, the jurists are unlikely to issue an outright rejection of the entire Obamacare program.

During the final days before the spring of 2012 kicked into gear, columnist Bill Frist wrote that "the court's decision could play a role in determining our next president."

In my opinion, as the nation's ultimate, "court of last recourse ruling body" the Supreme Court has a lot of leeway on what the majority of its nine members can and will ultimately decide. The many possibilities range from ruling on how much individuals and corporations can be required to pay toward health insurance, if at all.

The ultimate importance of this ruling grows in strength and importance when we realize that the court also might rule on everything from the amounts that physicians can be reimbursed to the amounts of benefits that patients are entitled to receive.

The court has final say, at least for the time being on this wide spectrum of Obamacare-related issues, or at least the widespread parameters that these issues entail.

Even so, you should always remain fully cognizant that whatever the court decides, at least in the short term anti-Obamacare advocates have the possibility of repealing the regulations—thereby making the jurists' decision moot.

Prepare for the Worst and Hope for the Best

The physicians, businesses and consumers of our nation should essentially "prepare for the worst but hope for the best" when anticipating the Supreme Court decision.

Under a worst-case scenario, a majority of the jurists could give a rubber stamp of approval to the entire legislation—opening up the floodgates for nationwide economic calamity as the overall size of the medical industry approaches one fifth of the economy.

The eventual ruling will come following open arguments heard by the court March 26-28, clearing the way for one of the court's most anticipated rulings of the past several generations. The ruling will decide the fate of suits filed against the federal government by 26 different states, plus various opinions that seven appellate courts have already issued.

Some analysts anticipate the court's ruling in June 2012, five months before the general presidential election, and about 18 months before Obamacare would begin forcing individual Americans to buy health insurance whether they want to or not.

Ultimately, the court will decide on the constitutionality of whether the government can require the purchasing of insurance— and also whether the Medicaid system, originally intended for only the poorest Americans, can be expanded to include about one out of every four Americans. Under current Obamacare regulations, certain people who refuse or fail to buy health insurance would be fined $695 per adult and $347 per child.

In addition, the court is likely to issue decisions on two side issues—whether the entire law "falls" or just part of it, if the jurists rule that part of the Affordable Care Act is unconstitutional. Putting spice into the drama, the court also will have the option of deciding whether it's able to rule on these issues at all—partly because Obamacare is not yet fully enacted.

James W. Forsythe, M.D., H.M.D.

Socialism Stinks

If the court approves Obamacare as passed by Congress, for the first time in our nation's history Americans will be forced by our federal government to purchase something.

Such a regulation would serve as a proverbial slap in the face to all of us Americans who cherish our freedoms, unfettered by a harsh or dictatorial federal governmental bureaucracy.

From my view and the perspective of many anti-Obamacare advocates, such a provision would threaten the entire U.S. free-market system.

After all, if the government is capable of forcing us to buy health insurance, what is to prevent the feds from forcing us to do such outlandish things as wear GPS satellite tracking devices or to wear tape-recorders devices around our necks at all times?

Sure enough, the very foundation of Obamacare could ultimately serve as the bedrock for lawmakers to gradually rob all Americans of our personal liberties.

Pushing the proverbial dagger into our hearts even further, the U.S. Congressional Budget Office has projected that individual insurance premiums might increase—according to various published reports—by up to 20 percent if the court clears the way for the Aact to go into full force and if we fail to rcpcal Obamacare.

"Politically, if the new law is judged constitutional, Democrats will celebrate the judicial affirmation of the spirit and substance of the historic reform—illustrating President Obama's leadership," Frist wrote in a March 2012 column. "Republicans would fan the existing flames of unpopularity among the majority of Americans."

Spin the Court's Ruling

Win or lose in this judicial round, all of us who oppose Obamacare can and should strive to remain positive, using whatever is decided to our advantage. We should follow these general tactics:

Unfavorable decision: If the Supreme Court approves

Obamacare, adversaries of the legislation should use the news to ignite the proverbial fires of political discontent. For the most part, conservatives successfully used this tactic about six months after the congressional approval of Obamacare—regaining control of the U.S. House of Representatives during the autumn elections of 2010. For the most part, many Americans are angry and mad at the U.S. government for forcing them to spend their own money, particularly expenditures on cumbersome federal programs. More than merely targeting Obama, we need to strive for ouster all U.S. Senators and congressmen who have supported Obamacare.

Favorable decision: When and if the court rules as unconstitutional some or all of Obamacare, we need to refrain from resting on our laurels. We must fight hard to oust Obama, largely because he would likely continue increasing the federal budget deficit if re-elected—while also striving as president to ram through more ill-advised medical industry legislation. Such a ruling also should motivate us more than ever to continue our quest for repeal.

Neutral ruling: If the court rules that it lacks the power and ability to issue any ruling until after Obamacare goes into full force, we need to use such inaction as a springboard to intensify our efforts.

Chapter 7

This Political Battle Will Last Many Years

We need to brace ourselves for an extended political battle on this issue, possibly stretching for many generations to come.

The overall process is equivalent to the war on terrorism, but only in the sense that these heated differences shall remain for well past the lifetimes of those fighting the health care battle today.

To help put this into perspective, remember shortly after the attack on America in September 2001, when then-President George W. Bush proclaimed that the war on terrorism would continue for generations to come.

As another prime example, think of the landmark 1973 U.S. Supreme Court decision in the case Roe vs. Wade which cleared the way for legalized abortion. Now edging into the fifth decade since then, the issue seems hotter than ever with liberals and conservatives continually at odds on this highly emotional issue.

Well, right here I choose to predict that whatever the current sitting U.S. Supreme Court decides on the nationwide entitlement health care issue, lawyers, politicians, liberals and conservatives will be arguing the issue for many years to come.

Certainly, toward the tail end of the current 21st Century and perhaps well into the following 100-year period the issue is likely to draw heated disputes.

Let's Secure a Positive Future

From this moment forward let us work collectively to set the proverbial stage, clearing a pathway toward a positive future in

American health care. An integral part of this effort will be to repeal Obamacare as soon as possible and start rebuilding from scratch. To do otherwise would be to put in place a recipe for long-term disaster.

Everything comes down to the fact that people, particular those of ultra-liberal political philosophies, will continually demand that they receive public health care—essentially for free. By embracing a "give-me" society, we'll rob people of their incentives to earn their right to medical care.

Such a system would, in turn, sharply curtail any semblance of a free-market system where professionals strive to give the best, most innovative, cutting-edge services and treatments possible.

Indeed, in the decades immediately prior to the launch of Obamacare proposals consumers began flocking to the best, most reputable hospitals and physicians whenever possible—particularly those that generated well-deserved positive reputations.

Yet overall health care costs soared high during the same period, largely due to excessive and unnecessary government regulations. Coupled with cumbersome requirements imposed at the urging of greedy Big Pharma, overall medical treatment costs soared much higher than average families could possibly afford.

This trend in turn contributed to the growth and power of health insurance companies, which in essence are legalized Ponzi schemes—particularly within the life insurance arena. Those huge firms essentially began using fees collected from some policyholders to pay off those who filed claims.

But the problem swelled as the overall medical fees zoomed much higher than lots of analysts had anticipated. This interlinked revolving door of continual rising insurance premiums eventually created a "snowball effect," where rising medical fees automatically sparked insurance premium increases. These two interlinking factors essentially began to feed off each other—as if fast-running, continually moving rats on opposite sides of the same treadmill.

James W. Forsythe, M.D., H.M.D.

National Health Care Consistently Fails Worldwide

Historians, politicians and sociologists have consistently warned that "history repeats itself," essentially a clarion call that society needs to learn from mistakes of the past and from problems experienced in other cultures.

Well, within the realm of national health care, virtually all such systems have emerged as dismal failures on an international scale.

To our nation's credit, at least until the advent of Obamacare the United States remained one of a handful of major, wealthy industrialized countries to avoid a blanket nationwide health care system designed to cover all people.

Prior to any rush to approve Obamacare we should have done more to patiently and effectively study problems plaguing those many failed or inadequate systems.

Invariably by rushing the legislation through to passage without any substantive discussion whatsoever, the U.S. Congress failed all Americans.

Use Other Failures As Examples

Any common-sense effort to carefully study the United States' health care issues should have taken into account the many criticisms and failings of these other countries' national health care systems. Among them:

Canada: According to various news reports and government studies, patients needing urgent or important medical care sometimes must wait many weeks to get confirmed appointments to visit physicians. In fact, according to a Canadian government report, the median wait time to schedule a physician visit is two weeks—and some unlucky patients nationwide need to wait up to 90 days to see a doctor. Worsening matters, once a physician in Canada schedules a surgery the average patient must endure a median wait time of a whopping four weeks before the operation, according to the same Canadian government reporting system. Some published reports even claim that common dogs—mere household pets—can get a hip replacement surgery in less than one week in Canada—while a person needing similar surgery sometimes must wait several years. The wide variety of other apparent problems range form restrictions on patient funding—essentially mandates requiring that a patient must be certified as uninsured before certain treatments can commence. The problem has gotten so bad that some frustrated Canadian patients have traveled to the United States to arrange their own medical treatments that they pay for—rather than wiggle through a maze of Canadian government regulations.

Japan: People who lack private health care as employees or as family members of workers can sometimes qualify for such services via local governments. Yet when certain expenses reach high levels individuals under the national health care system sometimes must apply for loans or subsidy applications in order to cover the expenses. Some analysts worry the financial burdens could last a lifetime, carried on to subsequent generations.

Switzerland: The national government provides compulsory regulated and universal coverage to every person who lives in the country, under the Federal Health Insurance Act of 1994. Although the system is "universal," all residents must pay for part of their own health care coverage, covered by an annual deductible fee. National law prohibits insurance companies from profiting off required basic health plans—but the firms can generate revenues from supplemental plans. To cover these expenses, the nation's citizens must pay up to a whopping eight percent of their personal incomes toward their insurance premiums. Adding insult to injury or illness, patients also must pay for part of their treatments.

Taiwan: Since its enactment in 1995, the compulsory, single-payer National Health Insurance system has drawn heated criticism. Although 97 percent of the population uses the system using "smart cards" to track their coverage, some observers warn that the government has found itself with no option other than to borrow from banks to cover the expenses—because the system fails to draw enough money from workers' incomes to cover overall medical expenses. According to some stories quoting Taiwan's health insurance reform advocates, the premiums are regulated by politicians—reportedly reluctant to impose rate increases that might spark the anger of voters. Meantime, other moderate improvements in pharmaceuticals, the bureaucratic medical system has made keeping up with advancing technology difficult, cumbersome or impossible. Shockingly, according to an article published by the University of California at Los Angeles in 2003, the average patient's visit to a doctor lasts only from three minutes to five minutes.

England: The National Heath Service, primarily funded by the nation's general tax system, is often criticized for failing to be proactive. Proponents hail the system as "free at the point of use," meaning that patients pay nothing for nursing, bandages, visiting doctors and various medical checks such as Cat-scans. Although the system lacks any need for tracking information for billing purposes, patients accustomed to pro-active U.S.-style medical care sometimes become frustrated. Perhaps the lack of competition robs England's overall medical system of a sense of urgency. Meantime, for the past several decades England's politicians have been locked in heated political battles focusing on expenses, patient care and the best ways to render such services. As a result, the politicians essentially are making critical decisions impacting overall patient care—primarily rules implemented by elected leaders who have absolutely no medical training or experience whatsoever. The overall situation got so bad at one point that the government launched an effort to essentially "modernize medical careers." But the implementation of this system got so bogged down that frustrated senior physicians nationwide eventually boycotted in 2007, according to BBC News. England's efforts at upgrading or modernizing its medical treatments got bogged down so badly in a bureaucratic maze that its national director, Professor Alan Crockard, submitted a resignation letter saying that he had "responsibility, but less and less authority." Adding to this bureaucratic mess, officials adopted mandatory "European Time Directive" hours, limiting the time that physicians could work. This generated criticisms that the poorly managed, government-operated system was essentially detrimental to patient care. And, as a result of the bureaucratic quicksand, there weren't enough surgeons to fill all shift rotations.

Chapter 8

Obama Ignored Top Experts

While pushing for his health reform in early 2010 Obama ignored official warnings that his plans would drastically increase the costs Americans pay for such services.

News reports issued in December 2009 quoted a Congressional Budget Office projection that Obamacare would generate average $2,100 annual increases in family premiums.

Obama either ignored or refused to acknowledge the numerous negative financial impacts that his plan would have on the typical U.S. family.

Thus, our anti-Obama political advertising campaign should boldly proclaim "the president's medical plan is ripping money right out of your pocket. To avoid getting ripped off, vote for the other candidate."

Adding to our political firepower, we can also stress that in the wake of Obamacare's passage chief officials for Medicare and Medicaid acknowledged that the measure would increase consumer spending on medical expenses by more than $311 billion through 2019.

Forecasts Rapidly Worsened

The official forecasts of Obamacare's upcoming damage worsened even further, when the Congressional Budget Office—sometimes called the CBO—updated the projected costs of the legislation to a mind-boggling $1.113 trillion. By some accounts, Obamacare's long-term financial expenses doubled by the time federal bean counters were able to re-estimate the totals in early 2012.

Obaminable Care ~ A Prescription for Chaos

"Even that estimate is low," Sally C. Pipes said in her eBook, "The Pipes Plan: The Top Ten Ways to Dismantle Obamacare."

Pipes, a health care industry expert, took the courageous stand of proclaiming Obamacare a dismal financial failure.

The Obamacare costs exceed $2 trillion for a 10-year period starting in 2014, including the expansion of Medicaid, health insurance exchanges and other costs, Pipes' publication says.

Based largely on these findings, packed with official government projections, I'm among a steadily growing number of physicians who agree with Pipes that Obamacare must be repealed as soon as possible.

The Prognosis ~ Gloomy and Worsening

Like Pipes has done in recent years, I've also been quick to point out that through the second decade of this century average annual health care costs will swell an average 5.8 percent.

Pounding proverbial nails even further into our flailing economy's coffin, as predicted by actuaries employed by Medicare at least one half of all medical expanses in the United States will be paid for by the federal government.

"This push for socialism is going to rapidly tear down the fabric of our entire economy, while destroying the whole medical industry," I tell anyone who asks me to explain these specific details. "People who understand this will get angry."

Adding fuel to the flames of discontent, we also should publicize Pipes' findings that "bending the cost curve in health care downward will be impossible without staving off Medicare's looming bankruptcy and staving off its long-term finances."

This mountain of problems will flatten the pocketbooks of future generations to come unless Obamacare gets stopped in its tracks at this early juncture.

"The outlook is, obviously, dismal and unsustainable," Pipes said. "But it's actually an optimistic take on the entitlement's finances."

James W. Forsythe, M.D., H.M.D.

Hospitals, Doctors and State Governments
Need to Worry

Various news reports, blogs and print publications do an excellent job reporting some of the most distressing details on these projections.

Several publications note that Richard Foster, the chief actuary for Medicare, said in his official report's appendix that the projections do not represent a reasonable expectation for actual program operations.

Among the most distressing key factors here hinge on projected Medicare savings that even Foster's report labels as an "implausible expectation." You see, those who crafted Obamacare legislation had envisioned cutting 2012 Medicare imbursement rates by 30 percent, slashing funds given to various health care providers including hospitals and physicians.

At least some of the problem apparently stems from the fact that Congress has been unwilling to raise rates imposed on seniors, thereby failing to keep up with rising medical costs.

Additional government reports project an inability to generate profit will strike at least one out of every seven health care facilities due to medical rate cuts mandated by Obamacare. The official forecasts expect a disturbing one out of every four such facilities will fail to reach profitability in 2030.

Patients and Health Care Operations Will Suffer

Although most people will have coverage through Obamacare, steadily increasing numbers of physicians, hospitals and health clinics will refuse to see or to treat them.

Simply stated, health care professionals would lose money by seeing the patients. Among primary factors that help put this into perspective:

Expensive: The average overall costs of treating individual patients would exceed the amount of promised or planned government revenues.

Competition: At least in some specific situations, patients who have expensive self-insurance policies will be deemed as "less cost prohibitive" to treat.

Worsening: The steadily worsening situation will feed upon itself, as if a festering, untreated and rapidly growing cancer. This mirrors my long-held person view that the worse the overall problem becomes, the less likely that potential new physicians or medical experts would enter the profession.

Permanent: Once Obamacare got entrenched deep in the American culture, there would be almost no way to fix the Act's many widening problems.

We'll Sink Faster than the Titanic

In essence, weighted down by Obamacare the entire U.S. economy is like the ill-fated RMS Titanic passenger liner that sank just more than a century ago.

Like the Titanic had been, Obamacare has many liberal supporters who foolishly declare it as "unsinkable," and the "greatest new innovation available to mankind."

Unless we take decisive action now, the vast majority of us within American society are "going down with the proverbial ship." Overall the U.S. medical industry will plummet into the depths of despair, a catastrophe far more widespread and severe than the Titanic disaster, at least on a broad scale.

Historians tell us that 1,517 people perished when the Titanic sank. By comparison, tens of millions of Americans would be left without adequate medical coverage, many of them unable to get any treatment or at least basic necessary care.

Please understand that in pointing this out I'm not trying to use excessive "scare tactics." As far as I know, there has been no formal estimate on how many consumers will die premature or otherwise preventable deaths due to Obamacare.

Even so, all the data that I've carefully reviewed on this issue clearly shows that huge swaths of society undoubtedly would suffer as a result. Would Obamacare doom hundreds of thousand or even millions of people to premature deaths? Would streams of people suffer debilitating physical pain or be forced to endure unnecessary or otherwise preventable disabilities?

As a physician who relies greatly on in-depth analytical studies and statistical analysis, I believe it's too early to issue official gloomy forecasts in this regard. Nonetheless, based on what I know about this destructive legislation, my heart and mind tell me that Obamacare would generate immeasurable human suffering.

Rather than fixing the nation's medical infrastructure and insurance industry, Obama's plan is slashing American health care infrastructure into irreparable pieces.

Millions Will Plummet

An estimated whopping 18 million Americans would remain without health care coverage at the end of this decade—even if Obamacare clicks into full force. That's according to official estimates by Medicare officials.

Foster has admitted that nearly 15 million people would lose medical coverage that their employers provide for them, as Obamacare adds 13 million individuals to policies.

"The whole mess is a wreck going into two different directions," I stress during presentations to physicians and patients. "At this point the only prediction that seems to have any credibility is that Obamacare would generate a maze of misunderstandings."

The Patient Protection and Affordable Care Act is tantamount to putting a baby-size bandage on a gaping, body-length wound suffered by a Tyrannosaurus Rex dinosaur. Fatal gangrene will set in unless the entire injury is sewn and covered in antiseptic gauze.

More precisely, Obamacare has already emerged as a scattered hodgepodge of "fix-it" efforts, never coming anywhere close to addressing continually increasing insurance premiums and health care costs.

The bureaucracy plans to continue to mandate cumbersome paperwork and record-keeping requirements for many types of medical coverage, while also mandating that insurance companies accept "all applicants" despite pre-existing medical conditions. That's tantamount to forcing a restaurant to give lavish all-you-can-eat meals to obese people, while forcing healthy, fit and trim people who exercise to pay everyone's bill.

Chapter 9

Beware of a Swelling Federal Bureaucracy

Remember, as passed by Congress, Obamacare would force all taxpayers to buy health insurance whether they want to or not—marking the first time in history that the federal government forces all of its citizens to buy something.

Various news stories and federal reports estimate the government will hire at least 16,000 new IRS agents to enforce this rule. Already labeled by bureaucrats under the politically correct term "individual mandate," a highly controversial section of the new health Act would severely penalize taxpayers who fail to prove that they have purchased health insurance for themselves and for their families.

When submitting their tax returns, citizens would be forced to include information proving that they have current health insurance policies.

Penalties for violators would increase from $95 or 1 percent of income, whichever amount is greater starting on January 1, 2014. Potential penalty amounts would gradually rise to $695 or 2.5 percent of income, whichever is greater, in 2016. Adding to the bureaucratic gook, the government will allow certain exemptions for cases regarding supposed financial hardship or for certain religious beliefs.

Like a majority of Americans as indicated by public opinion polling, I think this provision stinks. The very notion of forcing people to fork out their own money for this nonsense shows that we'll get what we deserve—a perennially inept government.

Angered by the selfishness of Obama and Congress, I agree wholeheartedly with the late President Ronald Wilson Reagan when he said: "Government is not the solution to the problem—government is the problem."

Health Insurance Companies Share the Blame

I'm among observers who complain that greedy health insurance companies have played a significant role in crafting legislation requiring people to buy such policies, as required by Obamacare. Among primary reasons for this greedy legislation:

Unhealthy people: As an overall industry, the health insurance companies feared that forcing them to accept people with pre-existing medical conditions would make their businesses either unprofitable or losing propositions.

Healthy people: In order to level the playing field, the insurance companies finagled lawmakers to force people considered healthy to acquire policies as well. This way, the corporations plan to generate enough cash flow to cover expenses of "unhealthy people."

Robin Hood Syndrome: This is in a sense the equivalent of the Robin Hood legend where someone "robs from the rich in order to give to the poor." The difference here is that people who take great care of their own health or those without pre-existing conditions such as hereditary ailments would be forced to essentially help "cover the bill" for people who overeat, refuse to exercise or unlucky enough to have hereditary diseases.

Rate-Raising Arguments: Insurance companies have argued that any failure to force "healthy people" to obtain policies would give their businesses no other option than to raise rates.

Public anger: According to a Gallup Poll issued in February 2012, an overwhelmingly high 72 percent of Americans—seven out of every ten people—consider the individual mandate forcing U.S. citizens to buy health insurance as unconstitutional. The same poll found that 47 percent of Americans want a Republican president so that the law can be repealed, an effort that 44 percent of respondents would oppose.

James W. Forsythe, M.D., H.M.D.

Seize Control of the Forced-Purchase Issue

Those of us who strongly oppose Obamacare need to make the "individual mandate" requirement of buying insurance a hot-button issue of the campaign.

Instead of generating expensive, difficult-to-understand TV commercials and radio spots on the overall health insurance reform—we need an easy-to-understand message.

Perhaps the best, most efficient way to accomplish this would be to air brief segments of "real people" describing their anger.

"I deserve to make my own health care decisions," a graying, middle-age couple would say. "How dare those bureaucrats swipe money out of my bank account to pay for their nonsense. If I wanted their worthless health insurance, I should be able to make that decision myself—not some bureaucrat."

Other than personal issues and all-out physical attacks, almost nothing makes a citizen angrier than the notion that big corporations or government is stealing from them.

Collectively and individually, those of us who oppose Obamacare need to essentially drive this point home as persistently and consistently as possible.

Liberals Spin These Arguments

Determined to muddy the proverbial waters, over-the-top liberals who strongly support Obamacare have argued that despite the mandate that insurance companies cover people with pre-existing conditions—those firms will strive to "chase away" the chronically ill.

The bottom line here is filled with nothing but worthless hot air.

On the flip side, those of us who despise Obamacare point out that if the government is allowed to force insurance purchases—"what is to prevent them from taxing people for being fat, or from forcing us to buy only products that are produced in China."

Indeed, the mere notion of enforcing all the senseless

gobbledygook in Obamacare has literally reached the point of stupidity.

Yes, we need to diligently and consistently work to give sensible updates to the existing tax code to benefit and motivate everyday consumers.

Add Benefits for Average People

Upon the urgent repeal of Obamacare, we need to diligently work to give consumers health insurance-related tax breaks similar to those enjoyed by huge corporations.

Just as important, in order to intensify competition and thereby generate lower rates, we need to allow people to buy health insurance from outside their own states. This would counteract repressive Obamacare policies which would require only in-state purchases of such policies, a process that stifles competition and results in higher rates.

Among other positive legislative improvements that I recommend after repealing Obamacare:

Health savings accounts: Improve tax benefits for such programs, giving consumers more incentive to set aside funds for future medical expenses anticipated as they age.

Expansion: Rather than increase the size of government or paperwork, add or improve benefits to consumers without increasing the costs to taxpayers.

Eliminate Senseless Requirements

The Obamacare regulations also would impose a maze of senseless requirements that some bureaucrats and even liberal journalists refer to as "mandates."

This term offends me and many other physicians and consumers; the word "mandates" seems to imply that these rigorous rules were imposed because an overwhelming majority of the public has demanded them or issued a clarion call that they be enacted. Proponents insist such a bureaucracy would level the playing field, making health care available to the masses on a far wider scale than ever.

To the contrary, however, streams of corporations will drop health care coverage altogether rather than cover the burdensome costs or relentless streams of required forms. This likely will leave many employees to fend for themselves while scrambling to obtain required but increasingly expensive health insurance.

Among my biggest fears here is that many people with good jobs will generate too much personal income to qualify for government assistance in obtaining mandatory health insurance. So, rather than face exorbitant IRS fines, many of these people will end up getting gouged by greedy insurers—leaving consumers with less discretionary income.

I worry that all these factors under Obamacare would play a significant role in dragging down the entire U.S. economy.

So, what's the solution?

It's simple. Besides repealing Obamacare, we need to essentially quarantine the American public—keeping consumers and taxpayers away from socialistic rules that would bog down the entire free-market system.

Allow the Marketplace to Generate Reasonable Rates

Pipes uses sound, clear reasoning when suggesting a solution to Obama's destructive and burdensome mandates. She urges that we "allow for a real health insurance market to develop with high-deductible plans coupled with deregulated health savings accounts."

This strategy will work, she says, because "getting rid of or significantly reducing mandates will make insurance more affordable and do more to move us toward a system of universal access to care."

Increasing numbers of medical industry analysts and conservative commentators began to embrace this overall view as the 2012 presidential campaign intensified.

By the time the election year finally arrived, streams of anti-Obamacare blogs and Websites appeared. All major Republican presidential candidates vowed to make repealing Obamacare among their top priorities as soon as they took office.

Meantime, at least from my perspective, the number of pro-Obamacare postings and sites seemed to pale by comparison. Only ultra-liberal, pro-Obama forces that yearn for a bloated, swollen U.S. government bureaucracy strived to champion such efforts.

Chapter 10

We Still Have Time to Win

"It ain't over till it's over," still hails as one of the most famous quotations from retired professional baseball legend Yogi Berra. This legendary line remains embossed in the American vernacular, a call for everyone to fight to the very end.

Fully embracing such a strategy, all of us who despise Obamacare need to realize and always remain cognizant of the fact that we can still "win."

Although Obamacare squeaked through Congress in early 2010, we should seize the opportunity to use the public's anger to bolster our cause.

The ultra-liberals who seek to tear down the fabric of America's competitive health care system would like us to believe that "the public is stupid, and that people forget." The socialists want to tell people how to live their lives, to dictate what is "good" for them.

Well, to that we say: "Balderdash."

"I'm mad as hell, and I'm not going to take this anymore!" People screamed this out of their windows in the hit 1976 satirical film "Network" starring Peter Finch. His character galvanizes the nation, imploring the public to express its discontent.

By comparison, judging by what I'm hearing in the hallways at hospitals, from patients and from doctors, people from many walks of life across our nation are frustrated by Obamacare and streams of them are downright mad at our president's loony political policies.

U.S. Supreme Court Decisions Sparked by Politics

Both conservatives and liberals realize that many of the most controversial U.S. Supreme Court decisions are politically motivated—rather than based strictly on the law.

Largely for this reason, Democrats and Republicans strived to force certain justices off the case in advance of the March 2012 hearings before the court.

The "Huffington Post" reported that conservatives strived to get liberal Justice Elena Kagan off the case. With just as much fervor, literals strived to seek court rulings to force conservative justice Clarence Thomas to sit out the case, the Post reported.

The publication said that neither justice budged at the removal efforts. The parties in the case never formally asked the justices to remove themselves.

"But underlying the calls on both sides is their belief that the conservative Thomas is sure to vote to strike down (Obama's) health care law, and that the liberal Kagan is certain to uphold the main achievement of the man who appointed her," the Post said.

Like many other Americans, while opponents and opponents of Obamacare argued the issue before the Supreme Court in March 2012, I worried that the jurists would base their opinion primarily on their own individual political ideologies.

Once again, this motivates me to re-emphasize the point that no matter what the court decides, Obamacare opponents need to remain energized to fight for our cause.

The Conflict Intensified

Political combatants also acknowledged that the difference of just one vote on the nine-member court could drastically alter these jurists' overall decision on Obamacare. Among their specific arguments:

Thomas: His wife Virginia worked for several firms that opposed the Act, leading liberals to call this a conflict of interest for which Thomas should recuse himself from the court's Obamacare hearings.

Kagan: Conservatives complained that while serving as the solicitor general for Obama she may have played a role in crafting Obamacare. Those seeking to pull Kagan from the case also wanted to know any opinions she gave on the issue before Obama appointed her to the Supreme Court.

"The campaigns against the justices are partisan, suggesting to some legal experts that the complaints are less about perceived conflicts than the outcome of the health care case," the Post said.

Federal law requires that any Supreme Court justice sit out of any case where his or her impartiality might "reasonably be questioned." However, this rule strikes me as silly and pointless because many decisions are obviously political anyway, and allegations of apparent impartiality are cloudy issues that almost anyone could allege at any time.

Acknowledge Extreme Challenges

The opponents of Obamacare need to fully acknowledge that repealing the legislation would be an extremely complex and challenging task.

Many of our allies would naively have us believe that any repeal of the Patient Protection and Affordable Care Act could occur via the stroke of a president's pen.

Early on in the 2012 presidential campaign all major candidates made it clear that they will strive to obliterate these regulations as soon as they move into the Oval Office.

Yet in order for our collective efforts to get the best results, all of us need to acknowledge that various roadblocks or hurdles would occur. Among them:

Executive mandate: Some candidates including former Massachusetts governor Mitt Romney vowed to issue an executive order upon taking office, excusing states from Obamacare requirements. But a maze of legal challenges would soon erupt.

Congress: In order to quickly sweep the repeal through Capitol Hill, conservatives likely will need a majority in the House and the Senate—plus a Republican in the White House.

Fully cognizant of these formidable challenges, GOP Congressman Steven Arnold "Steve" King of Iowa and Sen. James

Obaminable Care ~ A Prescription for Chaos

Warren "Jim" DeMint, a South Carolina Republican, jointly wrote an article in the conservative "Washington Times" entitled: "End Obamacare, Don't Mend It." The lawmakers wrote that Obamacare is even more unpopular than when it was foisted upon the public, and that it'll cost almost $2 trillion.

"The American people were told Obamacare would reduce health care costs, but premiums already are jumping," the King-DeMint article said. "The American people were told they could keep their own coverage, but a new Congressional Budget Office Report says millions will lose their current coverage every year."

The Monstrous Federal Panel

Throughout the 2012 campaign I shall continue to join the efforts of lawmakers such as King and DeMint, especially their strident warnings against a little-known panel created by Obamacare.

The 15-member Independent Payment Advisory Board, sometimes called iPAB, will be loaded with bureaucrats having absolutely no medical training or knowledge whatsoever. Among horrendous factors that come to play here:

Unelected: These officials will be unelected, never accountable to the public.

Cronyism: The danger looms that appointments to this panel will be made as political favors.

Accountability: Because board members will be accountable to no one except perhaps to politicians who appointed them, the danger looms that members will favor big business interests rather than consumers.

Knowledge: Although they lack medical training, these appointees will essentially make life-and-death decisions involving large segments of the public.

Powerful: Due to provisions within Obamacare, the board will be extremely powerful in approving or denying health care services within Medicare.

Short-Term Good News Hit the Airwaves

On March 22, 2012, four days before the Supreme Court's scheduled hearings on Obamacare, the U.S. House of Representatives voted to eliminate iPAB—essentially wiping out any chance that this ludicrous panel could ever get installed.

Yet for the eliminate-iPAB bill to become law, the legislation still would need approval by the U.S. Senate. Even then, following approval in both the House and Senate, the move to prevent iPAB from starting would face a potential presidential veto.

This loomed as a possibility. In the event of a veto, a vote by a two-thirds majority in both houses of Congress would be needed to override the president's efforts.

On the positive, from the prospective of anti-Obamacare advocates, additional good news emerged. Numerous Democrats expressed their displeasure with plans for iPAB, joining Republicans in voting to eliminate the panel.

However, as the Associated Press reported, the House vote had largely been symbolic: "The bill is likely to hit a dead-end in the Senate (which has a slim Democratic majority). House Republicans all but guaranteed that when they paired the board repeal with caps on Medicare malpractice awards, which most Democrats oppose."

Some Obamacare proponents have compared iPAB to "death panels," panels mandated by the regulation changes that some observers say would decide whether patients "would live or die." The liberal media eventually claimed that perspective of the panel had been debunked.

The iPAB board "is not necessarily a death panel, but it is a rationing panel and rationing does lead to scarcity for some," said Congressman Jack Kingston, a Georgia republican. "Who's going to get the needed treatment, an 85 year old or a 40 year old with children?"

Some House Democrats who opposed iPAB said they disliked the panel for different reasons than issues voiced by Republicans.

Obaminable Care ~ A Prescription for Chaos

The liberals supporting the elimination of the panel complained that the board would diminish the role of Congress.

An interesting analysis developed when some observers claimed that House Republicans actually wanted the Senate to eventually reject the iPAB-elimination bill. This way the Republicans would be able to make an issue of the panel in the campaign.

Bureaucracy Would Generate Inefficiency

Like growing numbers of physicians and other medical industry professionals nationwide, I'm concerned that the Advisory Board will concentrate too much on the money-saving aspects—rather than maintaining quality patient care.

"I'm afraid that everything will come down to these bean counters," I tell some of my closest friends and associates. "These bureaucrats on the panel don't know diddlysquat about health care. They're likely to bog down the entire medical industry."

Under the previous system being phased out due to Obamacare, a Medical Payment Advisory Commission or MedPAC had relied on policy makers and Medicare administrators. Their recommendations were sent to Congress for approval.

In a sharp contrast, the dangerous and overly bureaucratic iPAB will have the authority to make critical decisions—while Congress has authority to overrule these bureaucrats' choices.

The dangerous edge of the proverbial sword comes to play here largely because a primary task for iPAB will be to reduce Medicare spending—rather than fully focusing on improving health care and giving consumers freedom of choice.

From what I'm learning at medical industry conventions and within literature distributed to physicians, this panel likely will be more interested in minimizing costs than ensuring that the overall public has adequate health care.

Adverse Impacts on Patient Care

The primary stated objective of iPAB is to continuously concentrate on cost savings on a year-to-year basis. This is to start in January 2014, when the panel is designated to recommend its criteria for holding down costs in 2015.

Much of the process will hinge on continuous analysis on the effectiveness of current Medicare spending, coupled with future financial projections. But this process is tantamount to playing Russian roulette with the public's health. Among reasons:

Advancements: Sudden and significant improvements in health care often happen fast, while iPAB has little or no ability to quickly respond to such changes.

Cost changes: The costs of medical services and products fluctuate fast due to supply and demand, but iPAB would have little ability to respond in a timely manner.

Bureaucracy: Just one person, the Chief Actuary of Medicare, would be empowered to certify whether the iPAB recommendations would achieve certain cost savings.

Top Official: In the event that the Actuary declines to certify iPAB recommendations, the Secretary of Health and Human Services would have to submit a proposed method to achieve the proposed savings amount.

Congress: The secretary would then begin implementing the proposal, unless Congress decides to intervene.

If all this sounds overly confusing and too complex for you, then your thinking mirrors those of us who insist this puzzling maze serves as a recipe for disaster.

Political Nonsense Prevails

Those who support Obamacare might strive to point out that iPAB is strictly an advisory panel. While lacking full regulatory power, the board is to serve as an advisor to Congress. At face value, this might seem sensible. But a thorough analysis of these regulations reveals obvious flaws. Among them:

Congress: Our nation's top lawmakers have already screwed up health care enough. The notion of elected leaders making critical health care decisions is ludicrous at best.

Presidency: Under our form of government, the president has the power to veto any legislation. Thus, a politician with no medical training whatsoever could wipe out critical and essential health care systems, services or products with the stroke of a pen.

Focus: From my view, our legislative House, Senate and President should have more pressing day-to-day concerns and duties than to decide individual health care issues.

Legality: As if all these cumbersome factors did not already pose enough a problem, physicians, organizations or consumers likely would file lawsuits—complaining that too much or too little of specific proposals were implemented.

The Adverse Impact on Doctors

According to a May 2011 article in the "New England Journal of Medicine," the new system could occasionally cut Medicare fees received by physicians. This process was bad enough in the past, when Congress occasionally tinkered with physician fee schedules. The bureaucrats have strived to control Medicare's spending on physicians.

The American Medical Association has lobbied for changes in this "sustainable growth rate" method. The process occasionally had automatically lowered fees paid to doctors when expenses for previous years exceeded projected totals.

But Obamacare has already failed to overcome those flaws. Rather than generate "fixes to the problems," the Act will worsen billing and doctors' revenue issues.

This, in turn, likely will cause many physicians to stop accepting Medicare patients. Some doctors will avoid such people when revenues from those consumers fail to generate enough money for the physicians to cover their own expenses.

Once again, the American consumer will lose out due to Obamacare.

Beware of Senseless Bureaucracy

Each of the 15 iPAB members will be paid $165,300 yearly by the federal government, adding further to our nation's swelling budget deficit.

Worsening matters, if he wins re-election President Obama would have the ability to appoint the board's members for periods ending long after he leaves office. Thus, any subsequent conservative president immediately after he leaves office would have difficulty removing the entrenched bureaucrats unless Congress repeals Obamacare.

Under the staggering the members' terms, five members would have 1-year terms, five would have 3-year terms, and five would have 6-year terms.

While all this might sound logical at face value in order to stagger terms while retaining at least some cohesiveness, it means that Obama would able to pump up the panel with more of his cronies near the end of his second term.

Under the system, all 15 iPAB members are appointed by the president, who would make those decisions after consulting with the minority leader of the Senate, the Senate majority leader and the Speaker of the house. The speaker and the leader each would give separate recommendations on board members.

"As far as many physicians are concerned, the whole appointment process is a giant Category 5 hurricane headed straight in our entire industry's direction," I tell friends. "The costs of the upcoming damage will be immeasurable, lasting—I fear—for many generations to come."

A War of Words Erupted

Various bureaucrats and elected leaders have clashed in a media-driven war of words on the issue of the Independent Payment Advisory Board.

Opponents of Obamacare have reached the reasonable conclusion that generating this system is tantamount to telling innovative physicians and medical researchers that they essentially "cannot be in research anymore." Indeed, the bureaucratic maze would reach the point of absurdity under full-scale Obamacare.

From my perspective, the socialistic system championed by President Obama would be worse economically and less efficient than economic systems imposed on the Russian people at the height of that former superpower's communist regimes.

Essentially, Obamacare seeks to cripple the vital logistical process that would potentially make the entire U.S. medical system great if left alone. At this juncture, we need to understand that within the medical industry the science and art of logistics involves the efficient shipping, distribution and implementation of products, services and pharmaceuticals.

When unencumbered and unfettered in a free-market system, the entire medical industry could become highly efficient—while able to adapt to rapidly changing conditions and technological advancements.

To the contrary, however, the entire medical system is likely to bog down under Obamacare, like an ocean-liner resting at the bottom of the ocean—never to be lifted to sea level ever again.

Chapter 11

Envision the Horrors of Our Medical Industry Under Obamacare

Following several years of intense study, I have reached a shocking forecast on the future of the American health industry under Obamacare. Among negative outcomes:

Millions lose coverage: Many millions of people actually will lose their medical insurance coverage, because they or their employers are unable to pay rising costs.

Exodus: Streams of countless talented and experienced medical professional including doctors will eagerly exit the industry.

Languish: The ballooning of the medical bureaucracy will force patients to wait many months or even years for vital surgeries or basic medical appointments.

Closures: Streams of hospitals or medical clinics will close due to cost overruns, perhaps up to one out of every four such facilities.

Demand crunch: In many regions, particularly large metropolitan areas, the decrease in medical facilities will overload and overwhelm those services at remaining health treatment outlets including hospitals and clinics.

Personnel: Many brilliant people who once entertained the possibility of become doctors or nurses will begin deciding to avoid the industry.

Deaths and extended illnesses: An undetermined number of people will die due to inefficient medical care, while many others suffer extended or undiagnosed illnesses.

Flattened incomes: The sluggish and cumbersome system

bogged down by necessary paperwork will ultimately flatten and minimize salaries of doctors and nurses.

Lost incentives: The political and business quagmire will discourage the implementation of vital medical research that otherwise could benefit many people.

Untold suffering: Amid the slump in the overall medical industry, the overall life expectancy of Americans will continue to rise largely as a result of advancements in nutrition and cleanliness during the 20th Century. But although more people than ever will reach advanced old age, more of them will suffer due to bureaucratic medical maze.

Nursing home overload: The populations of nursing homes nationwide will swell to the bursting point. More than ever, people who eventually get into such facilities will be considered both "lucky and unlucky." On one side of the proverbial coin, they'll be lucky for getting into such a facility where they'll be looked after the rest of their lives. But on the flip side of this same paradoxical situation, they'll be highly unlucky as well—most forced to live in highly crammed environments, so densely populated that overall living conditions seem to become inhuman.

The Health Industry Will Impact All Aspects of American Life

To a great degree, the "human aspect" will be ripped out of the American medical system more than ever. Already gone, of course, for the past several decades was the era when general practitioners made frequent or at least occasional house calls—eras when just about everyone in a small town knew of and depended on "the doc."

By contrast, largely as a result of Obamacare, steadily increasing numbers of patients will start believing that they're "mere numbers" in the eyes of their doctors.

This is and will be a sad outcome, indeed, largely because the relationship between a physician and his or her patient can play an integral role in potential recoveries.

Sadly, however, under Obamacare our nation will become like other socialistic societies where government-run health systems become inefficient and highly impersonal As I've already noted, patients in some countries complain that they're essentially ground through the system faster than little pieces of candy zipped through a confection factory.

From other nations including countries in the Far East, I've heard horror stories of long lines of patients who each end up seeing their doctors for only a few minutes at most. And for that, those same patients pay taxes or contribute to medical funds.

Similarly, Obamacare is likely to drag down the overall status of the American medical industry to the level of a third-world country—and that's no exaggeration.

Consider Medicine on a "Human" Level

To help put this entire bureaucratic mess into perspective, I want to stress the primary reason why medical care is so important to many people.

On the basic level, everything comes down to the undeniable fact that modern medicine—and in many cases "natural medicine" as well—works.

Almost everyone knows that many drugs or natural remedies can lessen pains or relieve symptoms.

Thus, to intentionally force a patient to go untreated is to condemn that person to potential unnecessary suffering. Just as important, people who lack the resources to get necessary check-ups or treatments die much sooner than they would by receiving professional care.

Ultimately, of course, each of us will eventually die. As cooperative and highly intelligent individuals, for the most part humans have learned the importance of striving to help ensure that each person has a good quality of life.

All along, though, the issues of costs, resources and self-responsibility come to play. From political and philosophical standpoints, urgent questions erupt—namely, who should pay for medical care? What costs are reasonable? And, who should get the best service or medications available?

We Need to Face the Difficult Truth

As a society, as physicians, as medical industry professionals and as taxpayers, we need to collectively face a difficult issue.

The crux of the matter rests in the fact that not everyone can afford health care.

A huge percentage of people—at least half of all Americans by some accounts—will live in poverty at least for a time before age 65. In November 2011, the U.S. Census Bureau announced that in 2010 "median household income declined, the poverty rate increased and the percentage without insurance coverage was not statistically different from the previous year."

The cold, hard facts, at least when reviewed via the Census Bureau's unemotional press release, stated that the nation's poverty rate increased to 15.1 percent, up from 14.3 percent the previous year.

The Census Bureau did not use this word, but I'll say it here—a "whopping" 46.2 million people in the United States were in poverty in 2010. From my personal perspective, that's a huge number, especially when considering that more than 300 million people live in the USA.

During the same 1-year period, the number of uninsured Americans increased by nearly 1 million—reaching 49.9 million, up from 49.0 million the previous year.

Moral and Value Systems Come to Play

The politics, personal philosophies and religious beliefs become integral factors in determining the eventual outcome of Obamacare.

In many regards, the pivotal question comes down to this: As a society, and as a nation, should our government and ultimately the taxpayers be responsible for managing the health of the nation's nearly 50 million uninsured people?

Before I fully analyze this question and the many diverging potential answers, think of the following to put this situation into perspective. In an entire year, there are only 31.5 million seconds. Thus, under Obamacare as envisioned in a utopian society, every second our nation would have to pay for the medical needs of nearly two people.

At first glance these might seem like random, meaningless numbers.

But when taking into account data from the American Hospital Association the challenge becomes clear. The organization's published reports show there are just fewer than 942,000 beds in 5,754 hospitals nationwide.

In the event of a global pandemic that simultaneously sickens tens of millions of people in the United States, should society and our government equally fill those beds with people who will remain uninsured under Obamacare—and those who have self-paid insurance?

Under this imaginary scenario, half the beds would be filled with the uninsured and the other half would be filled by the insured. If and when such a tragedy eventually strikes as some experts warn, most hospitals would go so deep in debt that closing a majority of the facilities would become a possibility.

Due to sharply decreased competition throughout the medical industry, prices would soar as the overall quality of patient care becomes precarious.

Nagging Questions Will Persist

Throughout human history the question of how to fairly and equally treat the rich and the poor—if at all—has remained a heated and highly controversial topic.

Personally, I agree with historians and sociologists who list socialist, communist, fascist and totalitarian governments as dismal, utter failures in most regards.

Many of us argue that virtually all forms of government and political philosophies have serious flaws. Under communism Russia languished in a non-competitive system that failed to distribute efficient goods and services including medical care to the masses.

The Marxist ideology of supposedly treating everyone fairly and equally became a dismal failure. Fascist and dictatorial governments have proven just as repressive.

Meantime, for our part, the democratic and free-market system under capitalistic, competitive systems in the United States have generated problems as well. But from my view and from the perspective of many who join the fight against Obamacare, America's overall medical industry has consistently remained among the world's best.

Sure, prices for many medical products and services have soared far too high in the United States—not due to a lack of government regulation, but because of too much bureaucracy.

Move in the Right Direction

Basic human compassion demands that American society take decisive action to help the poor with medical care. But key questions remain, primarily at what cost and to what degree should taxpayers and those with good insurance policies pay or suffer as well?

The wide array of potential answers is as diverse as it is complex. Among the many intermixed factors:

Morals: Is it morally wrong to disrupt and damage the entire medical infrastructure due primarily to the effort to help the poor? Is it morally reprehensible to force many small and mid-size companies out of business, just so that the poor can get insurance?

Values: As Americans, are we willing to spend our own tax revenues for the express purpose of supporting a socialist government? Are citizens now barely scraping by to pay for their own health insurance willing to throw away the financial security and their grandchildren for the sole purpose of helping disadvantaged people get decent medical care?

When framed this way, these many questions help put into perspective that the overall issue of providing adequate medical care and insurance is not as easy as some people might want us to believe.

Some People Could Care Less

Adding to the complexity, we also need to face the fact that many people could care less whether our government fails, and lots of these individuals despise big corporations anyway. Many people are bitter against big government and huge business in the wake of the severe worldwide economic slump that intensified in September 2008, the loss of millions of jobs across the United States and countless home foreclosures,.

Nevertheless, as the spring of 2012 began, public opinion polls conducted by the Gallup survey organization indicated that Americans were more optimistic about the economy and employment prospects.

This scored at least some increases in President Obama's favorability ratings—which still remained low, under the 50-percent range. Many political analysts on both conservative and liberal TV networks concluded that those polling results did not bode well for Obama's re-election chances.

However, using history as a guide, the anti-Obamacare faction needs to remain cognizant that in the American political arena no one should ever underestimate an adversary. Underdogs can make resounding comebacks.

A key example of this occurred in 1948 when an infamously inaccurate "Chicago Tribune" front-page headline declared: "Dewey Defeats Truman." An iconic photo of President Harry Truman shows him smiling broadly while holding up the headline, proclaiming to the press: "This is one for the books."

Indeed, within the political arena sudden and unexpected

comebacks can and will occur. One recent example clicked into full gear when former Pennsylvania Senator Rick Santorum blasted into the top ranks of the GOP primary arena. At one point during late 2011 Santorum had no campaign office or staff.

Taking these classic come-back stories to heart, anti-Obamacare advocates need to realize that it isn't too late for us, that we can still storm to eventual victory.

Use the Values System as Our Rallying Call

We need to push the campaign to increasingly ferocious or even controversial levels.

A key strategy should involve spinning the morals and values dilemma into our favor, blowing the proverbial weather vane of America's mood into our favorable direction.

Certainly, we need to counteract the expected Democratic advertising propaganda that essentially will portray Obama as a saint sent from heaven to help the disadvantaged.

For this reason, we need to get to the forefront of this issue fast—essentially taking control of the morals-and-values issue first, and thereby making it our own.

Taking a lesson from the past, for instance, we might consider the type of controversial TV commercial that Lyndon Johnson used when campaigning to stay in the Oval Office in 1964 against Republican challenger, Sen. Barry Goldwater of Arizona.

A TV commercial promoting Johnson ran just once, featuring a little girl moments before nuclear Armageddon, and shocking many Americans into thinking that Goldwater actually would "push the nuclear bomb button" to launch a global thermal nuclear war.

Well, we can and should push for a simple, easy-to-understand but shocking TV spot that is just as likely to drive the morals and values issue home hard to Americans.

For instance, we could show a little girl crying upon hearing news of the death of her father, who lost his work-related health insurance due to Obamacare.

While such a tactic might sound stupid or asinine to some people, the strategy makes perfect sense when done with just the right tone. That's because evil-minded liberals will likely engage in similar tactics, but twisted to their own advantage. Envision an elated family shown because they finally get a "free ride," an all-expenses-paid ticket into a hospital at taxpayers' expense thanks to Obamacare.

Enlist Help from Physicians

Many Americans respect and admire doctors as an overall profession, even in the wake of continually rising health care costs.

Largely for this reason, we need TV commercials, radio spots, display ads and documentary presentations conveying the issue from the perspective of physicians.

I know first-hand from meeting with other medical professionals at many conferences in recent years that a vast majority of them strongly oppose Obamacare.

Riding on the strength of such discontent, our television ads could simultaneously show hundreds or even thousands of doctors disappointed with the legislative nonsense.

For added firepower, anti-Obamacare advocates must also consider putting streams of angry patients into these same ads or into separate advertisements.

Remember, this will be a propaganda war, so we need to essentially keep our opponents' expected game plan in mind at all times. The liberals will stop at nothing to muddy the issue, striving to confuse the public into believing a magic potion has emerged.

Chapter 12

Ignore Hogwash About Hope and Change

Many Americans fell for Obama's campaign hogwash about "hope" and "change" during the 20008 election season. At the time, he was the first major presidential candidate during that period to use this trashy tactic, but others including Democratic challenger Hillary Clinton followed suit—hoping to mirror or match his early successes.

But now after nearly four years of careful reflection, after striving to give Obama and his policies a chance, those of us who closely followed the health care issue realize there should have been little reason for hope about Obama—because he made things worse.

Any "change" that he might have brought about only created an unmanageable bureaucracy, while pushing up the nation's budget deficit to a staggering and destructive $15.5 trillion.

Anyone who cares deeply about our nation and for the welfare of future generations needs to understand and oppose the destructive nature of Obama's twisted policies.

In fact, the overall issue on the entire presidential campaign also comes down to morals and values, not just in matters relating to health care.

We need to ask the public: "Is it moral for the president to bankrupt you and your children as well? Is it against your values to cripple an entire segment of our economy, just so that a liberal president can satisfy his political cronies?"

Certainly, for the vast majority of Americans with average intelligence, the resounding and overwhelming answer to these queries would be "No." Thus, anti-Obamacare advocates need to stress this issue, not just in medical related issues.

Use Political Action Committees

American politics have gotten increasingly dirty during the four years leading up to Obama's re-election bid.

Lots of us vividly remember to our great disappointment the 2008 campaign when he promised to push through strong reforms in American political campaign regulations. Instead, Obama subsequently allowed political action committees to strengthen.

These organizations are able to collect obscenely high political donations, seemingly limitless contributions to push for political agendas. The political realm worsened in 2010 when the U.S. Supreme Court ruled that unions, corporations and individuals could give unlimited campaign contributions to Political Action Committees—commonly known as PACs.

Oddly enough, these regulations prohibit a particular political campaign from communicating its strategies and preferred messages with PACs that support the candidate's efforts. This way, greasy politicians can essentially "wash their hands" of any knowledge about political tactics or smear campaigns attacking their opponents.

Such hands-off policies could prove beneficial to a candidate if a political strategy supporting him backfires—thereby generating public controversy. PACs enable a candidate to deny any culpability or interaction in the greasy dealings of such committees.

Nonetheless, anti-Obamacare advocates need to donate and collect as much money as possible for PACs that support our cause. This is essential for many reasons. Among them:

Opposition: Labor unions that support Obama's over-the-top liberal policies are likely to amass a king's fortune in PAC donations. These funds, in turn, would be used to finance greasy, misleading ads that attack the eventual GOP presidential nominee.

Support: Pro-Obama PACs will crush our effort unless we amass huge piles of cash for our own Political Action Committees.

Timing: We need to launch our anti-Obama messages in a steady, well-timed manner as early as possible in the process in order to seize upon public discontent.

Chapter 13

Reach Out to Non-Partisan Voters

Our victory in the campaign arena rests largely on the decisions made by so-called "swing voters," mostly registered non-partisans likely to vote for either political party.

Various political polls that I have reviewed in recent years indicate that Obama's 2008 victory hinged largely on disenchanted, middle-aged voters—many of them white males. At a time when lots of them were discouraged by big business, Obama lied to these people—saying that he supported their cause.

But now I believe that many of these same non-partisan voters, both men and women, may consider themselves as burned by Obama's ultra-liberal policies, the runaway federal deficit and the growing ravages of Obamacare.

The anti-Obamacare faction must seize upon and help take advantage of this festering discontent to help ensure our victory.

Here is why some our most effective advertisements should feature actual disenchanted non-partisan voters angrily saying how they feel burned by Obama.

"The guy fooled me the first time around," one of our supporters might say. "But believe me, that man will never fool me or my family ever again. I would not vote for him if you paid me."

Use Networking to Convey This Message

Amid my work as a physician in recent years, I've heard steadily increasing numbers of patients and other health care professionals express their discontent with the president's policies.

These people feel like they were deceived and lied to by Obama

91

during the 2008 campaign and ever since. I live in Nevada, labeled by political analysts as a pivotal swing state that Obama visited numerous times during his first presidential bid.

That year, a majority of Nevadans who cast ballots favored Obama rather than his opponent, Republican Senator John McCain of Arizona.

Using such examples as a lesson, anti-Obamacare advocates need to concentrate on non-partisan voters likely to impact election results in swing states—where the margin of error in pre-election polling is less than 6 percent.

Political analysts tell me that high-populated, liberal states such as New York and California will vote for a Democrat presidential candidate almost every time. And numerous lower-populated Midwest or Southern states almost always vote Republican.

Thus, for us to help ensure victory we must capitalize on growing or festering public discontent in pivotal states likely to vote either way. To ignore these intense battleground regions would be to concede to our own eventual loss at the ballot box.

Public Petitions and Publicity

For many generations analysts have proclaimed that "all politics are local," even amid intense national campaigns.

Fully cognizant of this, we need to start grassroots state and national anti-Obamacare petition campaigns in the final months and weeks leading to the 2012 election.

Our forces and volunteers need to converge at popular regional and local public meeting places, such as grocery stores, shopping malls and churches. This will help increase our visibility and strengthen public support for our cause.

Conveying the message properly is also essential. To portray the correct image, our door-to-door campaigners should dress and behave as if average people, rather than wealthy, high-class Republicans.

When people see that many individuals from throughout their

communities support our political goals, the "undecided voters" might tend to empathize with or at least consider endorsing our cause.

For political campaigns, there is almost nothing stronger than to see someone you know or one of your neighbors campaign for an issue they strongly support.

Steer Toward the Middle

Although some analysts might sharply disagree with me, for any hope of victory the anti-Obamacare movement must steer toward the middle of the road.

You see, a vast majority of Americans typically vote for the candidate of their favorite political party, no matter what the specific issues. Estimates vary on specific percentages of the public that remain hooked to this criteria.

As an example, let's say 30 percent of all Americans always vote Republican and another 30 percent always vote Democrat. Under this scenario that would leave 40 percent of people who have a greater likelihood of voting either way. In essence, these middle-of-the-road voters are the people who will decide the outcome of the election.

At the same time, many of these same individuals dislike standard muddy politics. And, judging by impressions from media interviews, many voters shun people that they deem "too far to the right, or too far to the left."

Mindful of the essential need to carefully traverse this political minefield, anti-Obamacare should strive to avoid any images or wording that seems to portray all of our members or allies as being ultra-conservative or on the extreme right.

Certain political organizations such as the conservative Tea Party movement are likely to cringe at me for issuing such commentary. Whether we like to acknowledge this or not, many average Americans watching Tea Party advocates on TV will likely think of them as a bunch of "right-wing whackos."

Under this scenario, waving Tea Party Movement signs and shouting for the dismantling of our entire federal government is likely to offend or at least "turn-off" many middle-of-the-road voters. During the last few months immediately before the campaign started kicking into full gear, I started seeing sporadic news reports and Websites—all where Tea Party advocates blast Obamacare.

Rallies Generate Negative and Positive Results

Timed to coincide with the last few days immediately before the U.S. Supreme Court hearings on Obamacare, numerous opposition groups including Tea Party advocates were scheduling rallies in Washington, D.C. Steadily growing numbers of "Big-Name" conservatives had been lined up as the rallies' speakers, including former GOP presidential candidate Herman Cain.

As the political tensions mounted, I became increasingly concerned that widespread national and international news coverage of the rallies by the liberal media would use Tea Party images and comments taken out of context. This way, liberal journalists would strive to portray Obamacare opponents as idiots or at least wishy-washy individuals.

Certainly, in fighting the liberal health reform we should never be fearful of taking full advantage of the American free-speech system as granted by the First Amendment to U.S. Constitution.

All along, however, I'm among observers who strongly believe that the general news media as a whole carries a bias favoring the liberal agenda.

Meantime, highly conservative voters who attend such rallies should feel free to vibrantly voice their strong opinions on the issue. Yet they need to remain cognizant that for the most part at such events they're essentially "preaching to the choir."

Chapter 14

Join Medical Organizations for Support

We should seek the assistance and support of medical professionals in our political cause. Think of this as a primary way for us to breeze past any notion that anti-Obamacare is loaded with over-the-top conservatives.

Carefully following this strategy, all anti-Obamacare advocates should strongly consider making the Doctor Patient Medical Association a close political ally.

I strongly admire and appreciate the efforts of this essential organization, founded by physicians and patients who are strongly opposed to Obamacare.

This vibrant and increasingly powerful organization was co-founded by its chairman, Doctor Mark Schiller, an assistant clinical professor at the University of California, San Francisco—the same city where I attended medical school in the 1960s.

Besides his commendable and diligent work helping to lead the Doctor Patient Medical Association, Schiller is president of the Association of American Physicians and Surgeons. As stated in the Doctor Patient Medical Association that organization strives to achieve "freedom in medicine for doctors and patients."

As far as I'm concerned, such goals should continue to serve as the bedrock for those of us who want a sound, solid and reliable medical industry infrastructure nationwide.

Obaminable Care ~ A Prescription for Chaos

Let Us Strive for Individualized Patient Care

Rather than allowing the U.S. government to dictate when and how patients should be treated, we need to follow the lead of the Doctor Patient Medical Association. The organization clearly states in its literature: "Medical care is best when doctors and patients are able to make decisions together—We must strive to expand access to care."

Along this vein, the organization says, the decision on whether to participate in government programs should be left up to patients and doctors. Among the association's positions on other key issues:

Privacy: Doctors and medical professions should serve as a frontline defense in protecting a patient's privacy.

Freedom: Patients and medical professionals should remain unfettered from government requirements dictating medical care treatments.

Choice: Patients who choose to pay out-of-pocket, or who decide to remain uninsured should not be discriminated against.

Transparency: Doctors, hospitals and insurance companies should post prices so that patients can make informed decisions.

Competition: This creates a market for innovation, while also driving down prices.

Patient empowerment: Patients who are active, engaged and informed emerge as better partners in their individualized health care.

Take the "Common Sense" Approach

For the most part, all these various positions by the Doctor Patient Medical Association are complete opposites of Obamacare.

Throughout the process, unlike ultra-liberals who champion the president's health industry reform, the Association also stresses that each patient is different—with his or her individual needs.

From my perspective, it almost seems that if Obama had his way virtually all patients nationwide would be essentially "stuck on the same treadmill—everyone heading in the same direction but going nowhere, all using the same medicines and treatments."

Like many other physicians and patients as well, I find myself personally offended by such a notion. It's almost as if President Obama and the federal government all want to treat us collectively as either lab rats or operators of a prison.

Indeed, if I had an opportunity to calmly and rationally sit down face-to-face with the president to openly speak my mind on the issue, I would tell him: "Respectfully, I would like to tell you that your policies regarding medical care are flat-out wrong in almost every regard."

Obama's many allies like to romanticize the stories about how his late mother, Ann Dunham, would read him stories and school lessons. By almost every account, she must have been a bright, hard-working and delightful woman. With this clearly understood, I'm not trying to imply in any way that Dunham failed in her responsibilities as a parent.

However, everything about the man's socialistic tendencies tells me that something terrible had gone wrong with him somewhere. Any political policy or belief that is "too liberal or too conservative" borders on almost certain failure, just like Obamacare.

Love It or Leave It

Since American politics essentially remains a dirty, greasy process by design, anti-Obamacare advocates can and should consider conveying these messages:

Poor leadership: The president is a poor leader that has failed to accomplish anything significant while in office, other than to sign into law an act that will ruin the entire medical care industry—endangering the economy as a result.

Socialist: His socialistic policies favor people who want free, continuous handouts from the government—everything from medical coverage to school loans.

Budget deficit: The $15.5 trillion budget deficit created by the Obama administration will cripple the U.S. government and society for many generations.

Bad Choices: Rather than surround himself with advisors with moderate or even conservative views, his top staffers are all extremely liberal. Thus, he often fails to get sound advice covering a variety of political perspectives.

Courage: Obama lacks the courage to boldly say the obvious, loud and clear for all to hear: "The budget deficit is running rampant, out of control—and something must be done about it." Even liberal president Bill Clinton had enough gumption to acknowledge this during his own administration, before working to balance the 1990s budgets.

Fuel Prices: Remember, almost nothing will convince American voters to flee from a candidate than to learn that he or she "is pulling money from their pocketbooks." Seizing this opportunity, we need to make clear that per-gallon gasoline prices have soared more than $2 during Obama's first term, while he has done nothing significant to alleviate the problem.

Capitalize on Anger

Intensely angry at the Obamacare proposal, in October 2011 voters in all 88 of Ohio's counties overwhelming passed a referendum preventing the regulations from taking effect in their state. The "Weekly Standard" reported that statewide the measure won by 32 point, a whopping 66 percent to 34 percent.

Anti-Obamacare advocates nationwide need to capitalize on this still-burning discontent from coast to coast.

Almost every significant public opinion poll that I've reviewed on the issue shows that the American people hate the notion of this nonsense being forced upon them.

Keep in mind that despite passage of the Ohio referendum, such actions never could become law in any state. The permanent downside of such efforts emerges when recognizing that federal law takes precedence over state and local regulations.

Nonetheless, those helping to lead our worthy anti-Obamacare cause viewed the effort as a decisive psychological and moral victory. The "Cleveland Plain Dealer" labeled the referendum a "strike at President Obama's health care plan."

Use Ohio's Vote as a Positive Springboard

Wherever advance planning and time permits, anti-Obamacare advocates should launch similar statewide referendums nationwide for November 2012.

Even if Obama wins re-election, he would face a steep uphill political battle throughout his final four-year term in the event that voters in many or all states resoundingly proclaim their disapproval of his health care reforms. Such an outcome could emerge as likely, judging by public opinion polls that consistently show most Americans oppose the regulations.

Even many Democrat voters from Obama's party have resoundingly voiced their discontent with the policy.

In fact, in its early reporting of the 2011 Ohio vote, the "Plain Dealer" reported that the "measure was ahead by a wide margin in Cuyahoga County—a traditional Democratic stronghold."

Raising the hopes of Obamacare detractors, throughout 2011 and into the spring of 2012, many individual news reports chronicled growing public discontent. On the second anniversary of the measure in March 2012, the public seemed angrier than ever about the measure's congressional passage.

This "Poison" Could Kill Democrat Policies

In his "Washington Times" column published at the "Real Clear Politics" Website, Dr. Milton R. Wolf called Obamacare the "Kryptonite of American politics. Not even Superman himself could survive touching the truly terrible law."

Taking a clear, bold and strident stand, Wolf proclaimed that Obamacare is "heading for the ash heap of history, where it belongs, and so are the politicians who forced it upon an unwilling America. Good riddance."

A cousin of President Obama, Wolf is a board-certified radiologist. In a November 2011 column, Wolf argued that Democrats lied to the American people when pushing for the legislation's passage.

"They claimed that Obamacare would allow you to keep your current insurance and your doctor. False," Wolf wrote. "They claimed Obamacare would create 4 million jobs, 400,000 almost immediately. False. They claimed Obamacare would reduce the deficit. False. Their list of lies goes on."

Taking a strong and courageous stand, Wolf went on to report an undeniable, verifiable truth that Democrats undoubtedly never wanted him to reveal. As he succinctly reported, after the liberals lies began to unravel, they "shamelessly began granting Obamacare waivers to their closest friends."

These revelations sparked the ire of Wolf and many other sound-minded thinkers as well. Those of us concerned for America's future started questioning the honesty and devious tactics of the Democrats more than ever.

The Liberals Can Never Fool Us

Caught "dead-to-rights" as the old saying goes, the cunningly deceptive liberals pulled backroom shenanigans that made me and other flag-waving, patriotic Americans cringe. Their bold-face lies and mischievous behavior slaps all God-fearing U.S. citizens clean across the face.

As reported by Wolf and a stream of media outlets, the Democrats used the big-government machine to grant waivers to Obamacare regulations to at least 1,800 companies. Labeled by Wolf as essentially "get-out-of-jail-free" cards, these exemptions were the Democrat Party's way of thumbing its nose at the American public.

"We're going to stick it to the little guy, and to countless mid-size companies—while helping our buddies with favoritism," the Democrats must have been thinking to themselves. "Let's force average American to submit to this nonsense, while helping our closest allies skirt away from the nonsense that we created."

Among the major culprits cited by Wolf were House Minority Leader Nancy Pelosi, and Senator Majority Leader Harry Reid—both Democrats. Wolf complained that Pelosi "managed to carve out waivers for her fellow San Francisco luxury boutique owners."

Angered by such skullduggery, which should have been considered felonious in my opinion, in August 2011 the voters of Missouri paved the way for the similar Ohio ballot a few months later. Like those in the Buckeye State, the Missourians resoundingly passed an anti-Obamacare measure—in their case by a significant 3-to-1 margin.

Let the Democrats Hang Themselves

A keen researcher and analyst on the Obamacare issue, Wolf said flat-out: "Obamacare is the albatross Democrats have hung around their own necks. It's the curse of Ham, King Tut and the Great Bambino all rolled into one."

The president's own former head of Medicare, Dr. Donald M. Berwick, made controversial comments that seemed to blast Obamacare: "The decision is not whether or not we will ration care; the decision is whether we will ration with our eyes open. And, right now we're doing it blindly."

Berwick left his Medicare post shortly after he made this revealing comment, off script from the administration's political objectives.

"Dr. Berwick doesn't think much of you or your doctor," Wolf wrote. "He declares that the 'isolated relationship (between doctor and patient) is no longer tenable,' not without Big Brother calling the shots anyway."

Disturbingly, at least from my view, Berwick may have clearly stated the Obama regime's true but masked tendencies toward Marxism or even socialism. While still heading Medicare, Berwick said: "Any health care plan that is just, equitable, civilized and humane must redistribute wealth from the richer among us to the poorer and less fortunate. Excellent health care is, by definition, distributional."

Embracing the Shakespearean strategy of "kill the messenger," the Obama kingpins quietly booted Berwick from his post. Could the president and his various seedy rooks, knights and pawns have been irked that Berwick had publicly revealed that he favored the British National Health Service?

Wolf pointed out that at least 25,000 people in Great Britain die each year from unnecessary cancer.

"In many ways, Dr. Berwick personifies the arrogance that has permeated Obamacare, but that's not why he's hitting the bricks," Wolf wrote. "His cardinal sin, the one that cost him his job, is that he spoke truthfully of the Democrats' socialist agenda. The president denies that Obamacare rations health care or moves America toward socialized medicine, so Dr. Berwick simply had to go."

Romney-Care Plays a Major Factor

A 2012 Republican presidential frontrunner, former Massachusetts governor Mitt Romney, would likely complicate the issue as an eventual GOP nominee.

As the 2012 presidential campaign intensified, I would have been remiss by overlooking this integral factor. Under Romney's reign as its governor in 2006 The Bay State enacted a mandate requiring every resident of Massachusetts to obtain a minimum state-regulated level of healthcare insurance.

Muddying the issue from the standpoint of anti-Obamacare conservatives, streams of analysts insist there is essentially no significant difference between Romney's plan and that championed by the Democratic president.

Yet while striving to gain the nomination, trying to ally himself with Republicans nationwide on the campaign trail, Romney now vows that his first significant act as president would be to repeal Obamacare.

Thus, if Romney manages to scrape past hard-charging GOP challenger Rick Santorum, amid the final few months of the campaign Democrats likely would seek to portray the ex-governor as a dangerous and cunning "flip-flopper." Democrats would strive to make this work to their advantage, knowing that voters often shy away from candidates whom they perceive as highly wishy-washy.

Understandably, as reported in Josh Dzieza's March 2012 article for "The Daily Beast," Romney kept busy trying to distance himself from the Massachusetts law—"and no wonder, (because) the state and federal plans are virtually identical."

Romney Needs to Pull Himself Away

As an eventually Republican nominee, Romney would need to pull himself as far away as possible from the federal-state comparison. The liberally biased media likely would push this issue with relentless fervor.

"You can run, but you can't hide," slimy journalists would proclaim, striving to appear collegiate and highly intellectual. "As reporters, we're like former world heavyweight boxing champ Mohammad Ali, and, Governor, you're like his perennial challenger Joe Frazier—and we've got you on the ropes."

I recommend that rather than strive to dodge the issue or to spin questions on the matter in an obviously self-serving fashion, Romney should strive to go head-to-head against Obama on this steamy, highly controversial comparison.

"Romney-Care failed, and Obamacare will, too," the governor should say, creating a sound-bite that obviously will be used for many generations. "This is why I know perhaps better than anyone that Obamacare should be repealed as soon as possible."

When pressed hard to clarify further, as he surely will be, Romney should seize this opportunity to declare to Obama that "You're a socialist, sir—and that would tear down the fabric of our country. Mister President, why have you failed to state clearly that the runaway federal deficit will ruin our country?"

Obviously a crafty debater and a cunning wordsmith, Obama most likely will show anger that his patriotism has been questioned—careful to skillfully skirt the deficit issue.

At precisely this opportune moment, Romney would need to strike with a vicious, perfectly time and well-placed verbal sucker-punch. Whatever this crafty one-liner is, Romney should have it written and ready far in advance.

This seems necessary and quite possible. After all, any candidate such as Romney capable of spending many tens of millions of dollars campaigning during the early primary phase should be able to strategize and carry out such a plan.

I fear that unless Romney zips with heart, passion and fervor into such a directed battle, while also striving to "keep his cool" under the glare of the public limelight, he could soon find himself dipping deeper and deeper in pre-election public opinion polls.

Santorum Also Has Flaws

When heading into imminent battle, an army, a football team or almost any combatant needs to know its own many weaknesses and strengths.

Like Obama and Romney, the other Republican nomination frontrunner, former Pennsylvania Senator Rick Santorum, has his share of soft points and power spots.

On the negative side, at least from the perspective of many voters, Santorum might be viewed as by liberals and even non-partisans as essentially a "worthless far-right religious Christian fanatic."

Following years of America's involvement in wars in Iraq and

Afghanistan, many voters admit their wariness at the notion of any country or national leader steeped in religious fervor. Under this line of thinking, many of the world's bloodiest wars were the result of religious zealotry. Many adversaries undoubtedly carry such passion.

Still, from the eyes of many conservatives opposed to Obamacare, Santorum might seem far easier to passionately support. Following numerous victories for Santorum in several significant primaries, many Republican voters admitted that they had difficulty in trying to support Romney—whom many deemed as "not conservative enough."

Two months after primary voting began many voter surveys and public opinion polls indicated the public considered Romney "more electable" in a hypothetical one-on-one match-up against Obama. Nonetheless, Santorum marched to numerous victories in several states including Alabama and Mississippi.

One of my fears on the political front involves nominating a candidate such as Romney who fails to win the South in early voting. A presidential candidate deemed weak or unpopular in that region has less likelihood of reaching the White House, at least from the view of many seasoned political analysts such as the liberal Chris Matthews of the Democrat-leaning MSNBC-TV cable network.

Chapter 15

Amass Campaign Contributions at a Furious Pace

Many political observers predicted President Obama would collect close to an astounding $1 billion in 2012 campaign donations, far eclipsing the $670.7 million he pulled in during 2008. During his first presidential run, lots of those funds came from the so-called "little guy," individual voters who gave their donations via the Internet.

Adding to Obama's early advantage, marking him as a potential early frontrunner, as the 2012 race kicked into gear he was able to use his already-established emailing list generated four years earlier. Couple this with many millions of the president's Twitter followers, and within the realm of politics he would seem to zip faster than 1973 U.S. Triple Crown racehorse champion Secretariat.

On the positive side, Obama's re-election campaign spent money faster than it took in revenue as 2012 began. The "Boston Globe" reported that donors gave $29.1 million to Obama's campaign in January, down from $41.7 million during the same month four years earlier.

"USA Today" quoted Michael Malbin of the non-partisan Campaign Finance Institution as saying that "this is the first time the president's campaign has fallen behind its previous pace. Perhaps this explains the president's comments last week encouraging the activities of an independent super PAC (political action committee)."

Did Obama's slump in contributions happen because the president's support from non-partisans had weakened? If so, what could anti-Obamacare advocates do to take advantage of that apparent Achilles' heel—a term from Greek mythology signifying a deadly weakness despite overall strength.

With as much fervor and awe as possible, we need to attack Obama's political weak spot just as Achilles' adversaries did when shooting his heel with a poisoned arrow. To do this we must push public opinion in our favor by revealing Obama as a socialist.

House Republicans Jumped into the Fray

Republicans in the U.S. House of Representatives struck early, hard and with ferocity by re-introducing legislation in the spring of 2012—measures that the bill's sponsors said would move America away from a "dependent culture."

As reported by Fox News, "Democrats immediately blasted the plan as favoring big corporations over Medicare recipients."

The GOP plan for the U.S. government budget reintroduced a proposal first pitched in 2011, overhauling Medicare benefits for Americans who were under age 55 at the time that the bill passed.

Introduced by controversial Congressman Paul Ryan, the legislation would give eventual Medicare recipients from the under-55 age group options. These people would choose from a list of choices including private government-subsidized plans and fee-for-service plans that consumers pay to join.

Ryan, a Wisconsin Republican, said at a news conference that "we believe that competition and choices should be the way forward verses price controls that leads to rationing."

Some analysts were quick to point out that this hot-potato issue could emerge as a political quagmire for the eventual GOP presidential nominee during the peak of the fall campaign. Worries emerged amid some conservatives that uninformed voters would perceive the proposal as "forcing the little guy to pay more, while helping big business."

Conservatives need to teach voters that runaway government spending will cripple the economy unless consumers help to reign in the federal deficit. Yet telling the younger voters that they must essentially pay for financial mistakes of the older generation might tend to put a sour taste in their mouth.

As campaign rhetoric intensifies, Democrats likely will say that any taxpayer born on January 1, 1958, will have to pay big bucks for Medicare benefits—while any American born a day earlier on December 31, 1957, will essentially get a "free ride."

Simplify Issues for Voters

To emerge victorious we need to simply the issue into short, quick, easy-to-understand sound-bites in TV commercials and radio spots.

Our campaign needs to de-emphasize, ignore or shy away from any talk about consumers' out-of-pocket expenses. Instead, we must emphasize the need for people to have a choice—rather than deal with a shoddy, inadequate, pre-authorized government-mandated socialistic system.

Nonetheless, the top GOP contenders in all races from the presidency, to Senate and House positions should expect to get peppered with questions about their position on Congressman Ryan's measure. Many liberal journalists likely will spin their queries and reporting in such a way as to convey the incorrect message that "conservatives want you to spend more of your own out-of-pocket money for health care."

Fully cognizant of this potential quagmire, Gretchen Hamel of the right-leaning Public Notice told MSNBC-TV that she would "Tell them (Republicans) to support it. I think that they have a lot to gain by supporting a bold proposal."

Republican presidential contender Newt Gingrich, a former House Speaker from Georgia, had intensified the argument among Republicans in May 2011 after Ryan had initially introduced the proposal. At the time Gingrich called Ryan's plan: "right-wing social engineering."

Although Gingrich soon backtracked on those comments, the damage had already been done. This prompted Ryan to comment about Gingrich, "with friends like that, who needs the left."

Republicans Need to Stop Quibbling

Unless conservatives stop biting at each other's heels over petty political issues they likely will find themselves doomed to lose the 2012 general election.

Voters probably will shy away from any candidates perceived as unnecessarily bickering with or infighting with members of his or her own party. Certainly Democrats would seek to capitalize upon our perceived weakness here, our own Achilles' heel.

"There's a reason they call them (Republicans) the third rail in politics," said Eddie Vale, spokesman for Protect Your Care, a pro-Obamacare organization. "After the backlash they faced last year, even from Newt Gingrich, it's amazing that they're going to take another whack at it."

Appearing on the "Morning Joe" MSNBC-TV program hosted by conservative Joe Scarborough, Congressman Ryan said that the referendum will give voters a contrast to Obama's major spending programs.

"Let's give the country the choice of very clear two futures, let the people of this country decide in the fall and whoever wins the referendum gets to implement that plan," Ryan said.

From the onset I perceived the re-emergence of Ryan's proposal as a much-needed and welcomed Republican effort to make the many failures of Obamacare a penultimate campaign issue. This could "make or break" results for either party.

Chapter 16

Everyone Needs to Join This Cause

Anyone who truly cares about themselves, their families and the prosperity of the American job market should start opposing Obamacare. To put this into clear and concise perspective, thinking of this total—$25 trillion.

That's the Congressional Budget Office's estimate of Obamacare's unfunded liabilities through 2025.

The long-term health of your children, grandchildren and great-grandchildren will dip into extreme jeopardy due to the measure's regulation changes and funding.

Besides endangering the nation's economy, the measure also could put your own personal finances and health into severe jeopardy—especially for current adults.

Indeed, until my dying day, hopefully well past age 100 I shall remain vocal and vibrant in expressing the need for a competitive, full-bodied medical care system.

Now in my mid-70s, I often spend quality time reading with and playing with my three grandchildren along with my wife. As highly educated adults, as the matriarch and patriarch of our family, Earlene and I cringe at the notion that our increasingly socialistic government wants to squeeze very penny possible from these kids when they mature.

"President Obama is planning to rob your children," I tell some friends. "The man might think that his own heart is in the right place, but deep down he hates independent, free-willed thinkers who want to make their own critical decisions in life."

Stand Firm Amid Liberal Propaganda

To those just now joining our cause, or who have helped anti-Obamacare efforts for many months or years, I say: "Remain resilient. As the months and years pass, avoid falling for the hogwash and propaganda that the liberals will spew on this issue."

The long-term potential damage to our economy and to the long-term good health of all Americans is far too important to ignore.

Americans who avoid the issue or refuse to get involved politically likely will very soon regret their apparent indifference at this critical juncture.

By the grace of God, coupled with their own sense of decency and fighting for what is right, many people will join our cause in steadily increasing numbers.

I hope that you are among them.

Otherwise, all of us still living several decades from now could look back, telling ourselves: "I wish that I had joined the political fray. If only…"

Politically Pulverize Our Wounded Enemies

Obama used a "damned the torpedoes and full-speed-ahead" philosophy when ramming through his health care legislation.

His childish effort to push the untested scheme through Congress contrasted with his own consistent theme voiced during the 2008 presidential campaign.

Amid the final months of the highly contested Democratic primaries battles that year, the future president butted foreheads in the throes of his one-on-one skirmishes with his only remaining adversary, former First Lady Hillary Rodham Clinton.

Saying just about anything possible to trick voters, at the time Obama sharply blasted Clinton for her instance that health care reform should feature mandatory insurance. He also kept blasting Clinton for conducting her early 1990s medical reform efforts in secret.

Obaminable Care ~ A Prescription for Chaos

Yet desperate to shoot Obamacare through during his first 13 months in the Oval Office, he tacked on mandatory insurance and concocted back-room deals.

Obama "went wrong to unloading too much, too soon," former Pennsylvania Senator Arlen Specter, a Republican from 1965 to 2009, when he switched to the Democrat Party.

Sure enough, the president's reckless political leadership angered voters during the mid-term general election of November 2010. The electorate booted streams of Democrats from the U.S. House of Representatives in what many political analysts called the most significant congressional transition in more than six decades.

Emphasized his Warped Politics

We also need to stress to voters that when pushing Obamacare through, the president engaged in heated partisan politics—at a critical time when fixing the economy and addressing the federal budget deficit should have been his top concerns.

Overly eager to pin a political victory medal on his own chest, the president became more concerned with approving Obamacare paid little attention to specifics within his legislation. Among other key points to emphasize within the legislative realm:

Gridlock: The president's stubbornness and unwillingness to compromise on key issues created political gridlock in Washington, meaning very little got done.

Partisan politics: Obama's petty politics generated divisiveness as Congress failed to approve budget overrides needed to keep the government running.

Propaganda: A slow learner despite his crafty oratory skills, he concentrating on teaching the public to accept his warped politics. This marked a sharp contrast to former President Bill Clinton, who strived to work with his adversaries during his first term.

Lies: Essentially, Obama strives to convince Americans that they like his policies, especially his warped health care reform.

Adopt a "Scorched Earth" Approach

Our "scorched earth" strategy to take down Obama's political regime needs to bundle all his nonsense into one tight, neatly packaged, easy-to-understand bundle.

For added emphasis, we also can stress that at least early in the campaign the president and his warped allies were not out there actively boasting about Obamacare.

We never saw him taking a city-to-city national tour, telling everyone about the joys of his health care reform as the 2012 campaign clicked into full gear.

Romney, the front-running Republican challenger, rightly pointed out that "the White House is not celebrating Obamacare today." Truly, the public needs to know that the president kept hiding from this issue, as if hoping the debate would disappear. For many conservatives, the issue stemmed largely from the president's push for a huge federal bureaucracy.

"I'm going to return to the states the authority and the responsibility that states have always had to care for their poor and their uninsured," Romney said.

Emphasize the Puzzling Aspects

Increasing our firepower, anti-Obamacare advocates also should complain loudly and often that the legislation is seemingly even more complex than the IRS code.

Continually growing streams of corporate leaders and business analysts have started admitting that they fail to fully comprehend the entire legislation.

The puzzling regulations span from $2,000 per-employee penalty for any corporation that fails to offer health insurance. Analysts also warn that the costs that employers might pay insurance exchanges remains unknown.

Businesses and consumers also need to realize that health care prices covered by Medicare are likely to rise as the population ages.

To counteract the squeeze that Medicare incurs when extracting discounts from doctors and hospitals, those service providers are likely to start increasing charges to private insurers and employers.

Sharply increasing the bureaucratic complications, employers will be required to submit a maze of paperwork to the IRS. The Internal Revenue Service would then use that data to determine which employees are refusing health insurance. Adding insult to injury, the bureaucrats would decide if the workers are being offered inadequate policies.

Business Will Work For Government

I fear that more than any other federal mandate in history, Obamacare essentially will force all employers to essentially work for the federal government.

The required paperwork and communication by employers with their workers will rival or far surpass the regulations already imposed by the IRS. In fact, for the most part the federal tax filing and records keeping for annual returns is generally a matter of filling out required forms.

Much more disturbingly, Obamacare is likely to force employers to give continual updates to workers on available health care plans. Various blog postings and news accounts indicate that lots of human resources department executives worry that their divisions will get swamped with queries from confused and concerned workers.

The employees will be forced to choose from coverage at subsidized exchanges, a process likely to generate an unending stream of questions from workers.

"Everyone will want to know what is happing on a continually changing basis," I tell my political allies. "But the truth will emerge that in many cases few people if any will actually going on—resulting in chaos."

Essentially, the nation's federal tax system and its independent employers will become interlinked and mirroring each other. Like the famed Tweedledum and Tweedledee made famous in Lewis

Carroll's "Through the Looking Glass and What Alice Found," business and government will start looking and acting like each other in derogatory ways.

In the famed nursery rhyme Tweedledum and Tweedledee agree to engage in battle, but never launch such confrontation. Our government and industry essentially will be at each other's throats, always in the attack mode while accomplishing little or nothing.

Our Opposition Hates the Term "Obamacare"

The very use of the term "Obamacare" often disturbs our adversaries,

A column for the liberal "Washington Post" by Greg Sargent points out that the term "conjures up the ugliest images concocted by its critics: Obamacare is Big Government run amok; a threat to the American way of life; a symbol of all the ways Obama is scheming to deprive you of your liberty."

Yet Sargent quickly points out that the Act's proponents are striving to band together to use the label. On the legislation's two-year anniversary in March 2012, the Obama campaign sent its supporters an email saying: "It's about time we give it the love it deserves."

The epitome of hypocrisy, these creeps eager to spend your hard-earned tax dollars on government efficiency want to twist the truth to their advantage. Yet judging by the 2010 election results most voters including liberals refuse to fall for such deceptive tactics.

Hoping to confuse the issue, the Democrats will be saying for many years to come that "the public still does not understand the issue, because everything is just now beginning to take place." Hopefully, the majority of voters will refuse to get swooned into believing this nonsense, the line that "you'll love us once you know us."

Instead, we need to keep pushing the disturbing facts about Obamacare forward, rather than letting the Democrat's spin-machine rule the day.

Extra Extra

Victory Became Possible

Our potential for victory became apparent on the third and final day of the March 2012 U.S. Supreme Court hearings on the Obamacare issue.

The allies in our righteous cause had good reason to celebrate, when several news media outlets stated that the court signaled that the entire law might need to be eliminated.

All significant mainstream news media outlets reported that the entire health care reform act would be in jeopardy if the court struck down the provision requiring uninsured people to buy insurance.

"I think a majority of the court believes that if it rules that (the) individual mandate is unconstitutional, then the rest of the health care law cannot be saved," MSNBC-TV newsman Pete Williams said in his report after the court's final 90-minute hearing on Obamacare.

From my perspective as a frequent media observer on health-related issues, Williams' statement marked a significant concession by the highly liberal MSNBC.

In a seasoned and highly researched segment on the conservative FOX News reported the developments in bold and strident terms: "The nature of questioning over the last several days indicated several judges have serious doubts about the law. But they hardly indicated which way the often-divided court would rule, with a decision expected by summer."

Kennedy Plays a Pivotal Role

My intense, non-stop analysis of the ongoing court battle led me to believe that U.S. Supreme Court Justice Anthony Kennedy likely would serve as the pivotal swing vote—ultimately deciding the issue for the mostly divided court.

Kennedy asked lots of reasonable questions during the hearings that any sensible person should have been inquiring about. This increased my hopes that he would shoot down the selfish, ill-advised preferences of the court's four ultra-liberal justices.

The Obama administration had argued that if the court eventually decided to strike down mandatory purchases of health insurance, the justices should still guarantee insurance for all people while also keeping provisions designed to keep down costs.

However, as reported by Fox News, Justice Kennedy expressed concerns with such arguments. Using what anti-Obamacare advocates view as an ideal approach, Kennedy indicated that the situation might end up worse if all provisions of the law were retained.

"We would be exercising the judicial power if one act was stricken and the others remained to impose a risk on insurance companies that Congress had never intended," Kennedy said. "By reason of this court, we would have a new regime that Congress did not provide for, did not consider. That, it seems to me, can be argued at least to be a more extreme exercise of judicial power than to strike the whole."

Whiney Obama Bureaucrats Wiggled

Childish, selfish and self-centered Obama administration bureaucrats tried to muscle their plan through even amid Justice Kennedy's reasonable observations.

Those of us who know that Obamacare could destroy the fabric of our country cringed upon hearing reports on how Deputy Solicitor General Edwin Kneedler tried to ramrod a weak, scatter-brained argument on behalf of the administration.

Like a spoiled kid trying to get his way, stealing plates from other children at lunchtime in an elementary school cafeteria, Kneedler told the court that some provisions of the law had already clicked into gear—such as a regulation enabling adult children to go through their parents in acquiring health insurance.

"It's going to bankrupt the insurance companies," Justice Antonin Scalia interjected, clearly indicating that he was among jurists with a keen insight into Obamacare's persistent problems.

Giving anti-Obamacare advocates even more reason for hope, conservative Chief Justice John Roberts openly wondered "where is the fine line" as the court decides what to keep or omit from the act.

Force Government to Back Off

Ultimately, as reported by Fox News, for Justice Kennedy "the issue of compulsion raised concerns of whether the central government was getting too involved in peoples' lives." Observations such as Kennedy's landed dead-center at the heart of the bulls-eye on this issue, whether all law-abiding Americans should retain the right to make their own decisions.

Those of us who have closely followed the issue for several years wondered if the final day of the court's spring hearings on Obama care would essentially close the curtain on the "final act" of this liberal nonsense—or simply signal more arguments to come.

At the height of the controversy as the last of the three-day Supreme Court sessions closed, Chris Stirewalt of Fox News seemed to slam down hard on the Democrats' argument. Stirewalt penned his "Power Play" column under the headline: "Big Trouble for Obama if Court Creates Zombie Health Law."

By the time the hearings reached the third and final day, the individual mandate provision requiring people to buy health insurance was "looking very vulnerable," Stirewalt said. "The question of whether it can be severed from the rest of the law matters a great deal to the case. If it can be split out, the chances are higher that the key provision can be struck down. If justices decide that the law must stand or fall altogether, the stakes go way up for the litigants."

Remember these Keen Observations

Stirewalt's analysis and forecasts in the various potential outcomes of the Supreme Court's ultimate decision are worth noting. Among potential rulings and how he foresees the politicians to react:

Striking down the entire health law: During the election season, Obama would stress how "radical Republicanism" on the court has impacted the legislation. And having his one big achievement stricken by the court would be considered "a big embarrassment" for the administration. But amid proclamations by Obama's ultimate GOP presidential rival, Obama would "promise a better process in the future that would produce a better result." However, amid the ongoing debate from Stirewalt's view the arguments would shift from specifics to generalities, "always Obama's best subject."

Upholding the Law: For the president, winning could emerge as "worse" under this scenario. Although considered by liberals as a victory, this outcome could leave the president in a position where he needs to continue defending an unpopular law that was "crammed through Congress with procedural shenanigans." Meantime, a court approval of the law would galvanize anti-Obamacare advocates to the GOP nominee, thereby energizing the conservative campaign.

Keeping the law alive, while killing the mandate: Stirewalt believes that Obama would be in a world of trouble." The crux of the matter here rests in the fact that forcing healthy people to buy health insurance was deemed as a way to compensate insurance companies for being required to insure undesirable customers. This way healthy people and younger individuals would be forced to cover the costs of insurance companies' payments for those with pre-existing health conditions. But taking out the buy-a-policy rule would shatter the private insurance market. Stirewalt foresees that when and if this happens, huge premium increases would be followed by a loss of coverage.

Ultimately, Stirewalt said, for the Obama re-election campaign "a clear win or a clear loss can be dealt with, but nobody wants to deal with a zombie attack."

This Man Saw Through the Haze

Highly respected and seasoned political commentator Charles Krauthammer summarized the legislative controversy with grace and distinction. His comments mirrored those of us medical professionals who knew Justice Kennedy's pivotal role in the Supreme Court's ultimate decision.

Sparking the consternation of liberals, Krauthammer issued his comments on the Fox News "Special Report" with Bret Bair: "If you had left after the first hour (of the Supreme Court hearing) when the Obama solicitor general was being whipsawed and didn't have very good answers, you would have thought it was all over but the shouting, and that Obamacare was not going to survive. It was a rough hour for Obama's side.

But I think it was somewhat of a change in tone at the end of the second hour from Justice [Anthony] Kennedy, who essentially is the reigning monarch of the United States. He'll decide one way or the other what our future is going to be and what our Constitution is going to look like."

About the Author

James W. Forsythe, M.D., H.M.D., has long been considered one of the most respected physicians in the United States, particularly for his treatment of cancer and the legal use of human growth hormone. In the early 1960s, Dr. Forsythe graduated with honors from University California at Berkeley and earned his Medical Degree from University of California, San Francisco, before spending two years residency in Pathology at Tripler Army Hospital, Honolulu. After a tour of duty in Vietnam, he returned to San Francisco and completed an internal medicine residency and an oncology fellowship. He is also a world-renowned speaker and author. He has co-authored and written chapters in bestsellers. To name a few: An Alternative Medicine Definitive Guide to Cancer; KNOCKOUT, interviews with Doctors who are Curing Cancer and BREAKTHROUGH, EIGHT STEPS TO WELLNESS (Suzanne Somers' number one best sellers); The Ultimate Guide To Natural Health, Quick Reference A-Z Directory of Natural Remedies for Diseases and Ailments; Anti-Aging Cures; The Healing Power of Sleep; Outsmart Your Cancer: Alternative Non-Toxic Treatments That Work and Alternative Medicine Guide 2 Women's Health Series and "Compassionate Oncology" What Conventional Cancer Specialists Don't Want You To Know.

www.ingramcontent.com/pod-product-compliance
Lightning Source LLC
Chambersburg PA
CBHW072235290326
41934CB00008BA/1301